KILLING
ME SOFTLY
FROM INSIDE

KILLING ME SOFTLY
FROM INSIDE

THE MYSTERIES & DANGERS
OF ACID REFLUX

And Its Connection to America's Fastest Growing Cancer

—————————————— WITH ——————————————

A DIET THAT MAY SAVE YOUR LIFE

JONATHAN E. AVIV, MD, FACS

Book design by Tara Long/Dotted Line Design, LLC
Cover Art Design by Bobby Elijah Aviv and Tara Long/Dotted Line Design, LLC
Cover image ©shutterstock.com/Architecteur
Back cover photo by Richard Guaty
Interior photos: p. 10 ©CanStockPhoto.com/Pixelchaos; p. 201 by Nadia D. Photography

ISBN-13: 978-1494761974
ISBN-10: 1494761971

Library of Congress Control Number: 2013923458
Create Space Independent Publishing Platform, North Charleston, S.C.
Printed in the United States of America

To Caleigh, Nikki, and Blake
for their love and support

TABLE OF CONTENTS

PART 2 THE HEALTHY BODY   53

FOREWORD

It is a unique pleasure to author the Foreword to Dr. Aviv's ambitious undertaking to provide the public, as well as medical professionals in varied disciplines, with a comprehensive and insightful view of acid reflux, as well as presenting the reader with a practical dietary management strategy. I have collaborated closely with Dr. Aviv for over two decades while sharing many patients between New York and Boston. He is a dedicated and passionate physician and surgeon and deeply committed to enhancing the lives of his patients.

Dr. Aviv has been a key innovator in the diagnosis and management of reflux disease and has championed pioneering procedures such as TransNasal Endoscopy of the esophagus and Flexible Endoscopic Evaluation of Swallowing with Sensory Testing (FEESST). These diagnostic strategies are academically sound; however, these key innovations are disruptive to typical approaches and unduly remain at the periphery of mainstream practice. The resistance that Dr. Aviv has encountered is similar to my experience creating new philosophies and surgical treatment strategies for larynx (voice box) cancer and voice restoration. Consequently, we have had extensive discussions about approaches to creating the future by forging new management strategies in medicine and surgery.

His resolute determination has born *Killing Me Softly From Inside*, which is a passionate appeal to patients and the public to inform them about the silent masquerading detrimental impact of acid reflux and its implication as an important public-health issue. In an era when there are increasing institutional pressures to maintain the status quo, Dr. Aviv empowers readers with knowledge for them to enhance the "standard of care" rather than maintaining it.

Dr. Aviv's timely book weaves narrative patient and personal experiences with a scientific foundation that provides the reader with a valuable understanding of this substantial and expanding problem. This book provides a guide for individuals and patients for identifying, treating, and ultimately preventing the complications of acid reflux disease. Dr. Aviv introduces his Acid Watcher® Diet, which is an easy-to-follow meal plan to help treat the type of acid reflux disease that affects the throat, what he calls "Throatburn Reflux." The emphasis on using food as medicine is part of a growing trend for the future of healthcare and is exemplified in this enlightening and intriguing book.

Steven M. Zeitels, MD, FACS
Eugene B. Casey Professor of Laryngeal Surgery: Harvard Medical School
Director: Massachusetts General Hospital Voice Center

PREFACE

This book is written in two sections—*The Burning Body* and *The Healthy Body*. The first section, *The Burning Body*, explores the dangers of acid reflux disease, specifically Silent Reflux or, as I describe it in the book, Throatburn Reflux. This is a type of acid reflux without the noticeable symptom of heartburn. The concept of acid quietly, or softly, causing injury inside you, severe enough to be life threatening, is described with easy-to-follow tools and information. The intent is to help you identify symptoms that will direct you to seek proper medical attention early on, before the disease progresses to the fastest-growing cancer in America and Europe, **esophageal cancer**.

The second section, *The Healthy Body*, discusses what you need to do to achieve a healthy body by implementing a diet I developed called the **Acid Watcher® Diet**, which balances low-acid foods, proper macronutrients, and high fiber intake. This eating plan should keep you free of acid reflux disease as well as its unintended and devastating consequences. By following this diet, you should be able to both lose weight and maintain good health for many years to come.

Throughout the book, there is a recurring mini-section called the *Take-out Corner*. The *Take-out Corner* highlights key points and provides insight into strategies for avoiding and treating acid reflux disease.

PART 1
THE BURNING BODY

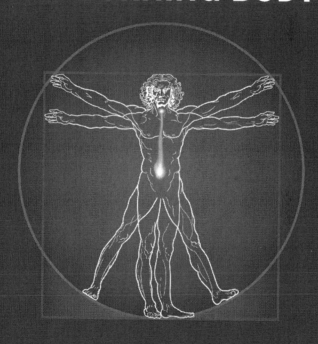

1

ACID REFLUX DISEASE—
THE MASTER OF DISGUISE

"I saw few die of hunger; of eating, a hundred thousand."
—BENJAMIN FRANKLIN

On a Friday night in October of 1996, I was suddenly awakened by the sensation of someone choking me. I couldn't breathe. The more I tried to inhale, the less air I could take in. I immediately started to panic. I was in my mid-30s and about to be married, with hopes of having children one day. As I gasped for air, my mind raced with fear. Was this how I was going to die—suddenly, in the middle of the night, with my fiancée sleeping peacefully beside me? *What was going on?*

I knew that I had only a few moments before I was going to pass out from a lack of oxygen to my brain. I had to do something. Instinctively, I compressed my lips tightly and started to slowly inhale through my nose, taking steady, deep breaths. This gave me the oxygen that my body craved. Thankfully, this steady, closed-lip sniff relaxed the spasm in my throat and the choking stopped.

So what had happened to me? At the time, I was the Director of the Division of Head & Neck Surgery at the Columbia Presbyterian Medical Center in New York. I was an ear, nose, and throat (ENT) physician and surgeon who specialized in swallowing disorders, as well as in perform-ing surgery to excise cancers of the head and neck. How could I, an expert in diagnosing and treating throat and breathing problems, have nearly suffocated in my own bed without a single warning sign?

I soon learned the startling reason for my choking episode. It was due to a form of acid reflux disease that rarely presents itself with tradi-tional symptoms such as heartburn and regurgitation. *How could I have had acid reflux but no heartburn?* Even my personal physician wouldn't accept this as a possibility. "It's got to be something else," he told me, "after all, you've never complained about having heartburn!"

Unfortunately, he was wrong. But luckily, my disease turned out to be reversible at the stage it was diagnosed. This frightening experience started me on a path of recognizing the otherwise overlooked, almost invisible symptoms of acid reflux disease in patients who were attending my own clinical practice in New York. Since then, I have seen and treated thousands of patients with acid reflux disease who, like me, didn't suffer from heartburn or regurgitation.

Throughout my career, many patients have asked me to explain to them what heartburn and regurgitation really are. Heartburn is best de-scribed as a burning sensation in the bottom of the chest and ribcage that can expand into the middle of the chest area toward the throat. Regurgi-tation, the other typical symptom of acid reflux disease, is the sensation of food coming back up into your chest and throat after you've already swallowed it.

Remarkably, over 90% of the patients in my ENT practice who are diagnosed with acid reflux disease do not have these typical symptoms. So instead of heartburn, they experience a sensation that's more like *throatburn,* along with other symptoms related to the throat, nose, sinuses, and lungs, such as cough, hoarseness, frequent throat clearing, a lump-like sensation in the throat, and regurgitation of stomach contents *into the throat*. They may also sometimes suffer from post-nasal drip, choking, and difficulty breathing.

This was so far removed from the conventional understanding of acid reflux disease that patient after patient would ask me, "Dr. Aviv, if I don't have heartburn, how could I possibly have acid reflux disease?"

I also noticed that many of the patients who came to see me had gone years without an accurate diagnosis, even though they had similar middle-of-the-night choking episodes as I had experienced. Some of my patients called these nocturnal choking episodes "jump-ups," because they suddenly jumped up in bed, gasping for air.

Generally, patients do not consider symptoms such as meal-time coughing, morning hoarseness, or excessive throat clearing dangerous enough to warrant a doctor's visit. However, when patients do visit a doctor, they are usually treated for allergies or asthma if they don't complain of heartburn. When these treatments don't bring relief, most patients simply think their symptoms are something they need to tolerate or a by-product of getting older.

At this point, you might be wondering what the big deal is with a little acid reflux, especially if there's no heartburn. The answer is that uncontrolled or poorly controlled acid reflux disease, whether accompanied by heartburn or not, could result in a pre-cancerous condition that can eventually lead to esophageal cancer.

Take-out Corner

Uncontrolled or poorly controlled acid reflux disease, whether accompanied by heartburn or not, could result in a pre-cancerous condition that can eventually lead to esophageal cancer.

The good news is that being aware of the non-typical symptoms of acid reflux disease enables you to take control of this part of your health care. Moreover, by becoming knowledgeable about non-typical acid reflux symptoms, like the one I experienced, you give yourself the opportunity to detect pre-cancerous changes in the esophageal lining before it may become cancer. The bad news is that most cases of esophageal cancer are detected too late, when the patient already experiences difficulty in swallowing because of a cancer blocking the esophagus. At that point, the cancer will have already reached an advanced stage. Regrettably, the average five-year survival rate at this stage is only 10-15%.

THE DRAMATIC RISE OF ACID-RELATED ESOPHAGEAL CANCER

Before 1970, esophageal cancer was attributed predominantly to smoking and alcohol abuse which resulted in a specific type of cancer known as *squamous cell carcinoma*. However, in the last 40 years, a different type of esophageal cancer, known as *adenocarcinoma*, has grown more predominant.

The incidence of esophageal adenocarcinoma was just four cases per million in 1975. By 2008, it had grown to an unprecedented 26 cases per million. This represents a 650% increase in incidence, making esophageal cancer the fastest-growing cancer in America and Europe. During this same time, nearly all other cancers (e.g., breast, colon, prostate) have remained flat or decreased in incidence (see Figure 1).

The main reason for the dramatic shift from one type of esophageal cancer to another is a result of the radical change in the American (or so-called Western) diet since the 1970s. Since that time, the profound prevalence and instant availability of large quantities of highly processed, very acidic, extremely addictive, unhealthy foods such as pre-packaged meals, salty, fatty snacks, sugary sodas, and coffee, have become so much a part of our daily lives. These ominous and horrifying "food" trends have been detailed by investigative journalists such as Michael Pollan,

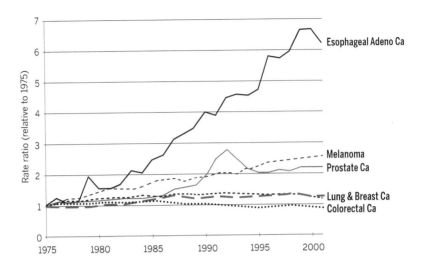

Figure 1 Rising Incidence of Esophageal Adenocarcinoma. Ca=Carcinoma. Pohl, H. & Welch, H. G. The role of over-diagnosis and reclassification in the marked increase of esophageal adenocarcinoma incidence. Journal of the National Cancer Institute, 2005. 97(2). 142-146, by permission of Oxford University Press.

Mark Bittman, and Michael Moss, as well as physician Robert Lustig, and chef and educator Anne Cooper.

The Western diet and lifestyle have completely taken over our health. Fast food, fast eating, caffeine-induced thinking, fast communication, fast, fast, fast! We do everything fast in order to keep up with the demands of our more and more complicated lives. We have become so demanding of ourselves that there are just not enough hours in the day to satisfy all that we need to accomplish. Thank God, however, we have the ability to get an incredibly strong cup of coffee on every street corner in every major city in the United States, so we can stay alert and in a state of constant emergency, every day, all day!

A special thanks, of course, should be bestowed upon the food industry that so compassionately tells us that they will save us a lot of time with instant this, instant that, packaged this, packaged that. We just have to open the box, microwave for 30 seconds, and there is our delicious, nutritious meal of the day! There is a meal for Daddy, a meal for Mommy, and even one for the baby— with a special toy in it!

But the gift of giving doesn't end with a toy. Chronologically coupled with our national dietary changes that began in the 1970s was a little-known federal law called Title 21. This law, enforced by the Food and Drug Administration (FDA), calls for the maintenance of high levels of acid as well as other additives in prepackaged foods to allow for a long shelf life as well as to kill any bacteria that might otherwise creep into the beautifully packaged food overflowing our supermarket shelves. In fact, there are 333 FDA-approved additives that have been added into our food. The health-safety decisions on how these additives are used has been left up to the food manufacturers, lacking any strict oversight by the FDA.

The prevalence of processed foods in our diet in conjunction with the consequences of Title 21 has created the ideal climate for our current acid reflux epidemic, setting in motion a perfect storm of conditions for the rapid growth of esophageal cancer.

DIGESTING THE FACTS

Most, if not all, foods in a can or bottle are almost as acidic as our own stomach acid. How does that affect our digestion? Consider for a moment that the stomach produces gastric juices that are very acidic in order to break down our food. The stomach does this in amounts that are proportional to how much food we eat. But what happens in the stomach when highly acidic food gets added and mixed in to our existing pool of stomach acid? The stomach starts to overflow with an excess of acid, resulting in this caustic substance flowing backwards and upwards out of our stomach into the adjacent esophagus, causing injury to our esophageal lining.

"So let me get this straight, Doctor," you might be asking right about now. "Are you saying that before the Western diet became more prevalent, and before that Title 21 law was passed to better preserve food, most people diagnosed with esophageal cancer got it as a result of smoking too much, but now most people that get esophageal cancer have it because of *too much acid going up into their esophagus?*" The answer is an unequivocal "yes."

Sounds shocking, right? Of course it is. Acid reflux disease has turned into an epidemic. Estimates are that over 50 million Americans have reflux disease without even realizing it. What has developed over the past 40 years as a result of this perfect storm of diet deterioration and legislative intervention is not only rapidly increasing acid-related esophageal cancer, but marked increases in incidence of obesity, diabetes, and heart disease.

To better understand how stomach acid could possibly get to the throat, the next chapter gives an overview of the anatomic relationship between the stomach, esophagus, and throat.

2

THE STOMACH IS CONNECTED TO THE THROAT

"Of several remedies, the physician should choose the least sensational."

—HIPPOCRATES

Believe it or not, the stomach is pretty small between meals, about the size of a fist. However, it expands slightly when eating and grossly expands when overeating. This is why we have to sometimes loosen our belts during or after a meal. The stomach is connected to the throat via the esophagus, or *food pipe*. This physical connection means that a problem occurring in the throat can be a symptom or consequence of a problem that actually started in the stomach.

A brief look at the anatomy of the esophagus will help you better understand the stomach-throat connection.

Let's start by visualizing the esophagus as an upright sausage that connects the stomach to the throat. This "esophageal sausage" is closed or squeezed off at the top and bottom ends with two areas of narrowing muscles known as sphincters. The Upper Esophageal Sphincter (UES) is at the top end, near the throat, and the Lower Esophageal Sphincter (LES) is at the bottom end, near the stomach. When we eat, the esophageal sphincters relax and open accordingly, allowing food to pass through the throat and down into the stomach.

What's crucial to understand is that in order for food to pass from the throat into the stomach, both esophageal sphincters must temporarily relax. As soon as the food passes through these muscles, they must tighten back up. In other words, this healthy functioning of the UES and LES allows food to pass only one way, and that way is down south (see Figure 2.1).

Figure 2.1 **Relationship of the Upper and Lower Esophageal Sphincters to the Esophagus and Stomach**

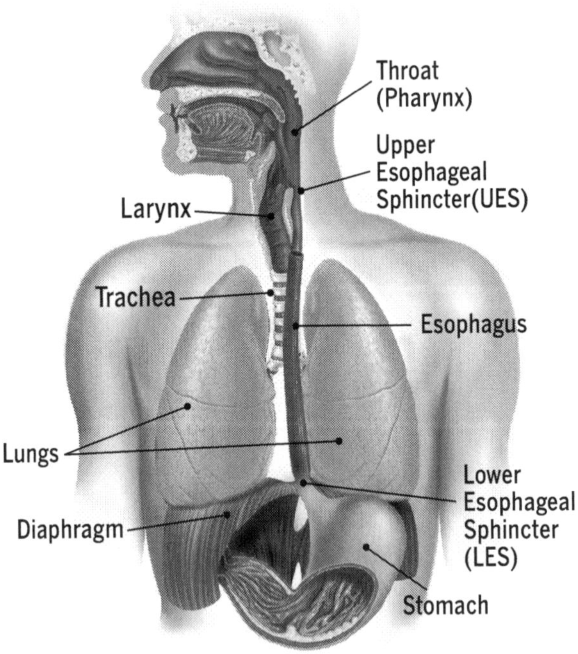

Note that the esophagus connects the throat to the stomach and is kinked at both the upper end, the UES, and at the lower end, the LES.

When the **LES** is not functioning properly and doesn't tighten back up after food passes from the esophagus into the stomach, the acid from the stomach can backflow into the esophagus, resulting in esophageal irritation. When the esophagus is irritated, one can experience a burning sensation in the chest, commonly referred to as heartburn. The term "heartburn" doesn't mean an actual heart condition. It simply refers to the fact that the pain resulting from acid injury to the esophagus emanates from an area adjacent to where the heart sits *anatomically*. This condition is referred to as GastroEsophageal Reflux Disease (GERD).

When the **UES** is not functioning properly and doesn't tighten up after food passes from the throat into the esophagus, stomach acid can travel all the way up into the throat, spilling onto the vocal cords and even into the lungs. This condition has been commonly referred to as LaryngoPharyngeal *(Lah-ringo-fehr-in-jee-ehl)* Reflux (LPR).

LPR can be quite dangerous because the throat, unlike the esophagus, is extremely sensitive to acid exposure. Studies have shown that even a single episode of acid hitting the throat can transform the vocal cords from thin, delicate vibrating structures into thick, log-like structures, which in turn can cause cough, hoarseness, and other throat symptoms (see Figure 2.2).

So what causes the upper and lower esophageal sphincters to loosen up? There are several reasons for the sphincters to malfunction. Among the most common are

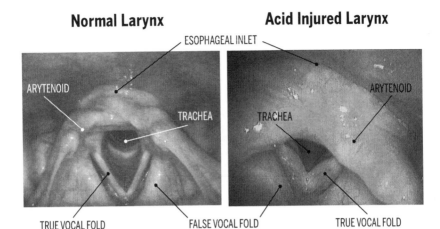

Normal Larynx

Acid Injured Larynx

ESOPHAGEAL INLET

ARYTENOID

ARYTENOID

TRACHEA

TRACHEA

TRUE VOCAL FOLD

FALSE VOCAL FOLD

TRUE VOCAL FOLD

Figure 2.2 Comparison of a Normal Larynx with an Acid Injured Larynx. In the normal larynx, one can easily identify the entire length of the vocal folds. In addition, there exists a space between the **true** vocal folds and the **false** vocal folds. The **true** vocal folds are attached to the back of the larynx by structures called arytenoids. The arytenoids are located at the back portion of the larynx, right near the esophageal inlet, or esophageal opening. Normally, the space between the right and left arytenoids are etched like the faces on Mount Rushmore.

In the acid injured larynx, one can only see the front half of the true vocal folds. The back half is "hiding" underneath the swollen arytenoids. The space between the true and false vocal folds is obliterated because the vocal folds are now very swollen. The area between the arytenoids has become puffy and ill-defined. In fact, that region now overhangs the trachea or airway. As a result, the airway is narrowed by almost half, compared to the normal appearing airway seen in Figure 2.2. Note how close the windpipe (trachea) is to where the food enters the esophagus (esophageal inlet).

widely consumed acidic foods such as caffeine, chocolate, alcohol, mint, spicy foods, and soda, as well as high-fat content foods. In addition, onion, garlic, and smoking loosen the esophageal sphincters, as does lying down right after you eat.

EVEN BABIES AREN'T IMMUNE

Several years ago, I suffered a traumatic event that clearly illustrates the concept of the stomach-throat connection. It involved my youngest daughter, Nikki, who was only eight days old at the time. During Nikki's mid-morning bottle feeding, she suddenly started choking and turning blue. I immediately called 911.

Fortunately, on the way to the hospital, Nikki's color returned to normal and there was no further choking. When we arrived in the Emergency Room (ER), her lungs and throat were examined and were found to be normal. She was then given another bottle, which she consumed without incident. After several hours of observation in the ER, Nikki remained stable and was discharged home. The ER pediatrician felt that this was simply an accidental choking episode and that we shouldn't worry.

Over the next few days, we noticed that Nikki had a raspy, hoarse cry coupled with a rumbling sound resembling an idling Harley Davidson coming from her chest. Nikki's pediatrician diagnosed her as having bronchitis, and she was prescribed the first of several rounds of antibiotics. However, the medicine didn't seem to help Nikki at all. In fact, after several months, her voice seemed to be getting worse and the chest rumbling continued.

TYING IT ALL TOGETHER

During this time, I was invited by the Mayo Clinic in Rochester, Minnesota to present a series of lectures regarding two related medical specialties of mine—acid reflux disease and swallowing disorders.

After my final lecture, the one on acid reflux disease, I chatted with the Mayo Clinic's remarkable pediatric ear, nose, and throat specialist, Dr. Dana Thompson. I told her about my daughter's choking episode and how she subsequently remained severely hoarse with a noisy chest in spite of having been given multiple courses of antibiotics for bronchitis.

To my surprise, Dr. Thompson turned the tables on me.

"Dr. Aviv," she asked, "do you really think your child is suffering from chronic bronchitis? Do you want to know what I think she's suffering from?"

"Acid reflux?" I asked sheepishly.

"Absolutely," she replied. "Even babies aren't immune to laryngeal reflux disease."

Upon returning to New York, I called Nikki's pediatrician and mentioned the possibility that she might be suffering from laryngeal reflux disease, or LPR, and not bronchitis. I asked that Nikki be started on an antacid medication in dosages appropriate for an infant.

"I'm willing to learn something new," the pediatrician responded. "However, let me run this by the head of pediatric gastroenterology (GI) at Columbia Presbyterian Hospital first. I'll get back to you."

Two hours later, my daughter's doctor agreed to start her on a three-month course of an antacid medication called Zantac (also known as ranitidine). Within six weeks, Nikki's voice improved, her chest noise disappeared, and she finally sounded as clear as ever.

This episode demonstrates the vital connection between the stomach and the throat. Even though Nikki suffered for several months with chest and voice problems, the real culprit was a distant organ—the stomach. Specifically, it was **stomach acid** being aspirated into her lungs during eating that led to her condition. Aspiration is defined as the inhalation of any substance such as saliva, food, or stomach acid sliding through the vocal folds, into the windpipe, then into the lungs (see Figures 2.1 & 2.2).

Unfortunately, the concept of the stomach-throat connection is often confusing to my patients. For example, Andrew, a healthy, active 37-year-old patient of mine with a penchant for diet soda and coffee, suffered from hoarseness, just like my daughter Nikki. He never complained of heartburn. After examining Andrew, I di-agnosed him with LPR and prescribed a low-acid diet and antacid medication. I further explained to Andrew that it would take somewhere between 6 to 12 weeks for his symptoms to improve.

Three weeks later, Andrew called me, sounding very concerned.

"Doctor," he said. "It's been over two weeks and I'm not better at all!"

"Andrew, are you taking the medication I prescribed?" I asked.

"No. I never started the medication. You gave me a stomach pill, and I need something for my throat!"

After I reiterated to him the connection between the stomach and throat, Andrew agreed to start taking the medication and to modify his eating habits. Within several months, his hoarseness disappeared.

Andrew represents about 25% of the tens of thousands of patients I have seen over the past 22 years who initially doubted the diagnosis I gave them because the stomach-throat connection, as detailed above, does not make intuitive sense to them. However, once the treatment regimen was followed, their symptoms usually improved.

Now that some basic anatomy and physiology has been reviewed, let's take a closer look at the phenomenon of LPR.

3

SILENT REFLUX: IT'S THROATBURN, *NOT* HEARTBURN

*"When you find yourself on the side of the majority,
it's time to pause and reflect."*
—MARK TWAIN

Patients such as Andrew who suffer from LPR generally do not feel heartburn because the effect of acid refluxing into the adjacent esophagus is so strong that, over time, it effectively numbs the esophagus so no pain is experienced. This is why LPR is often referred to as Silent Reflux, meaning the absence of heartburn.

However, I find the term "Silent Reflux" very misleading. It was initially coined to describe LPR based on the absence of only a single symptom (heartburn). But Silent Reflux is anything but silent because the heartburn symptom is replaced with a slew of throat symptoms such as cough, hoarseness, a lump-like sensation in the throat, swallowing difficulty, and/or throat burning. Therefore, I've come up with a term that highlights the symptoms patients actually experience. This more descriptive and accurate term for LPR is **Throatburn Reflux** (see Table 3.1). In

Take-out Corner ◥
Heartburn Reflux (GERD) presents in the chest area, while Throatburn Reflux (LPR) presents in the throat region.

addition, I've begun to refer to GERD as **Heartburn Reflux** as it is associated with the symptom of heartburn (see Table 3.1). These two terms give us a clear distinction between the two different types of acid reflux disease and their symptoms. **Heartburn Reflux** (GERD) presents in

the chest area, while **Throatburn Reflux** (LPR) presents in the throat.

Patients and physicians often disregard throat symptoms that would otherwise lead to proper diagnosis and care. They forget that the stomach is connected to the throat and instead cling to "good old heartburn" as the only possible symptom pointing toward acid reflux disease (see Table 3.1). In a sense, the absence of heartburn results in the absence of an accurate diagnosis. *Understanding that heartburn is not a symptom of Throatburn Reflux (LPR) is the single most important step towards developing an effective esophageal cancer prevention strategy.*

In order to focus attention on highly neglected throat symptoms, as well as a way to track responses to treatment, every patient who comes into my office is asked to complete the Reflux Symptom Index (RSI) (Table 3.2). It's a simple questionnaire that quickly assesses risk for Throatburn Reflux.

FEESST (Flexible Endoscopic Evaluation of Swallowing with Sensory Testing)

The idea that acid can numb tissues, in addition to searing them, is a very important concept. While I was at the Columbia Presbyterian Medical Center in the early 1990s, I invented a device called **FEESST** (**Flexible Endoscopic Evaluation of Swallowing with Sensory Testing**). It's an office-based, non-X-ray-requiring procedure that enables clinicians to measure sensation in the throat and to evaluate swallowing problems. FEESST is primarily utilized in patients with stroke and chronic neurodegenerative diseases such as Parkinson's, ALS (Amyotrophic Lateral Sclerosis or Lou Gehrig's Disease), MS (Multiple Sclerosis), Myasthenia Gravis, and the muscular dystrophies.

FEESST allowed me to demonstrate that acid injury from Throatburn Reflux (LPR) could cause enough swelling of the laryngeal tissues to result in numbness in the throat and esophagus. When a person's throat is numb, they are more likely to cough, choke, and aspirate. As a result, a person who notices that their symptom of heartburn has suddenly and inexplicably gone away without treatment should hold off before celebrating. In reality, the disappearance of their heartburn could mean that their acid reflux *is so severe* that their esophageal lining has completely lost sensitivity and they cannot feel the burning anymore, even though the damage is still present.

I want to make it clear that the source of both Throatburn Reflux and Heartburn Reflux is the same—acid from the stomach. One of the primary ways to make the actual diagnosis of acid reflux disease is to see signs of inflammation in the esophagus and top part of the stomach during

an endoscopic exam of these areas, which I detail further in Chapter 5.

Table 3.1
Throatburn Reflux Symptoms (LPR) vs. ## Heartburn Reflux Symptoms (GERD)

Throatburn Reflux Symptoms (LPR)	Heartburn Reflux Symptoms (GERD)
▶Hoarseness	▶Heartburn
▶Frequent throat clearing	▶Regurgitation
▶Acidic taste in the mouth	
▶Globus sensation (feeling a lump in the throat or that something is stuck in the throat)	
▶Trouble swallowing	
▶Chronic cough	
▶Aspiration (food or saliva going into lungs)	
▶Waking up at night due to burning in the throat	
▶Waking up at night with a choking sensation	
▶Excessive mucus in the throat	

Table 3.2
Reflux Symptom Index (RSI)

A score of greater than 13 strongly suggests that the patient has Throatburn Reflux.

Within the last MONTH, how did the following problems affect you?
(0=no problem; 5=severe problem):

Hoarseness or problem with voice	0 1 2 3 4 5
Clearing your throat	0 1 2 3 4 5
Excess throat mucous or postnasal drip	0 1 2 3 4 5
Difficulty swallowing food, liquids, or pills	0 1 2 3 4 5
Coughing after you ate or after lying down	0 1 2 3 4 5
Breathing difficulties or choking episodes	0 1 2 3 4 5
Troublesome or annoying cough	0 1 2 3 4 5
Something sticking in throat or lump in throat	0 1 2 3 4 5
Heartburn, chest pain, indigestion	0 1 2 3 4 5

TOTAL _____

Reprinted from Journal of Voice, 16(2), Belafsky, P.C., Postma, G.N., Koufman, J.A. Validity and reliability of the reflux symptom index (RSI), 274-277, 2002, with permission from Elsevier.

BARRETT ESOPHAGUS

Unchecked, acid reflux can lead to a disease known as Barrett esophagus. This is a potentially *pre-cancerous* condition typically appearing in the area where the lower part of the esophagus joins the stomach.

A normal, healthy stomach has an intense pinkish color, like smoked salmon or lox, while the esophageal lining has a grayish-white color. Generally, the pink stomach lining begins where the grayish-white esophagus ends. However, when there is severe acid injury to the bottom portion of the esophagus, the stomach lining starts to creep up into the esophagus, resulting in finger-like projections of pinkish tissue jutting into the grayish-white esophageal lining.

Barrett esophagus, or the presence of stomach tissue in the esophagus, is a dangerous sign for patients. It places that individual at a higher risk of developing esophageal cancer. In fact, those with Barrett esophagus are 30 to 125 times more likely to develop esophageal adenocarcinoma than the general population.

Barrett esophagus currently affects roughly 1% of adults in the United States. Men typically develop Barrett twice as often as women, and it is most common in white males over 50. However, over the past 10 years, I have been seeing men and women in their 40s, 30s, and even some in their 20s with this condition. Just last year, a 29-year-old patient referred to me with cough and hoarseness but *without heartburn* turned out to have Barrett esophagus.

Take-out Corner

Barrett esophagus is the presence of stomach lining where it shouldn't be, that is, in the esophagus. Incredibly, up to 15% of patients with Throatburn Reflux may have Barrett esophagus.

It is important to note that 8% of patients with Heartburn Reflux (GERD) may have Barrett esophagus. Ominously, 10–15% of Throatburn Reflux (LPR) patients, those who have *no heartburn* but do have chronic symptoms of cough, hoarseness, lump-like sensation in throat, and throat clearing, may have Barrett esophagus. By "chronic symptoms," I'm referring to symptoms lasting longer than eight weeks.

WHEN REFLUXED ACID REACHES OUR LUNGS

Have you ever thought that what goes on in your stomach can also affect your *lungs*? The fact is, the stomach, in addition to being connected to the throat, is also physiologically connected to the lungs. As a result, this stomach-lung connection may be the underlying cause of recurrent pneumonia or exacerbation of asthma in some patients. How does this happen?

In addition to allowing us to produce sound, our vocal folds are the major protector of the entrance to our lungs because they sit on top of the trachea, or windpipe. Even if a tiny amount of stomach acid reaches the vocal fold area, the vocal folds will reflexively close to protect the lungs. However, if a large amount of acid comes up from the stomach, it can overwhelm this airway protective reflex. Stomach acid will end up in the windpipe, or even worse, fall right into the lungs. This type of reflux episode can happen to anyone. As you might remember from Chapter 1, it happened to me while I was asleep.

I see this particular form of Throatburn Reflux several times a week in my practice. It is safe to say that almost all lung diseases are made worse by the presence of insufficiently treated or untreated acid reflux disease.

> **Take-out Corner**
> Almost all lung diseases would be helped by the control or treatment of acid reflux disease.

Refluxed gastric acid can cause a lot of damage beyond the throat and lungs. Even your tooth enamel, sinuses, or middle ear cavities can be affected by refluxed acid.

In fact, it is not rare for stomach acid to be found in the paranasal sinuses during sinus surgery or in the ears during ear surgery. It has been shown that both sinus and ear diseases can be helped by treatment of acid reflux disease.

The next chapter takes a more in-depth look into the relationship between cough and Throatburn Reflux.

4

COUGH IT UP!
COUGH AND THROATBURN REFLUX

*"Healing is a matter of time, but it is sometimes
also a matter of opportunity."*

—HIPPOCRATES

It would shock most people to know that one of the most misinterpreted symptoms in the history of medicine is cough. It is such a common symptom that it is considered mundane, even innocuous. However, I can assure you that it is not, especially if we are talking about *chronic* cough, or a cough lasting longer than eight weeks.

You probably never associated cough with acid reflux disease, but after reading this chapter you'll probably think of acid reflux disease every time you hear someone coughing. This happens to me all the time. I hear someone coughing constantly in the theater and I think to myself, "Has that person been checked for acid reflux disease?" I'm not talking about a cough related to a common cold or flu. I'm talking about a chronic cough, as further explained with the story below.

RIGHT PLACE, RIGHT TIME

A few years ago, I was flying home from a voice workshop I had guest lectured at in France. Sitting next to me was a lovely couple in their early 50s named Bob and Liz. We started chatting, and they shared details about their recent adventures in Paris.

About a half-hour into our flight, Bob started coughing. The more he tried to stop himself, the louder the cough became. It probably didn't help that nearby passengers turned to look at him, clearly wondering if Bob was going to disturb them for the rest of the seven-hour flight.

He went to the bathroom numerous times to try and cough up some phlegm, yet upon returning to his seat, his cough continued. Over the course of the flight, Bob explained that he had seen three different medical specialists who had sent him for multiple tests, including X-rays and allergy tests, but his stubborn cough remained. I asked him if any of his doctors considered checking him for acid reflux disease.

"What's the point?" he asked. "I don't have heartburn."

We talked about his diet and medical history. I found out that even though he was taking medicine for asthma for the past 10 years, his cough persisted. I suggested he speak to his doctor about the possibility that he might have acid reflux disease, specifically Throatburn Reflux. Maybe he didn't need asthma medicine at all. If Bob had any further questions, I recommended that he make an appointment to see me in my office so I could examine him thoroughly.

A few months later, I received an email from Bob letting me know that he followed through with my suggestions to be evaluated for acid reflux disease. His primary doctor referred him to a GI doctor, who

---

Take-out Corner

Cough is the most common reason patients see a doctor in the United States. It is responsible for 28 million patient visits per year, more than twice the incidence of the next most common complaint, headache. *It is one of the most misdiagnosed symptoms in medicine.*

performed an upper endoscopy that revealed esophageal inflammation consistent with acid reflux disease. He was treated with antacid medications, and his cough improved somewhat, but not completely. I suggested, as long as his personal physician did not disagree, that he begin a regimented low-acid diet program that I would put together for him. Three months later, not only was his cough almost completely gone, but he no longer needed to take asthma medication.

Almost one out of every 10 Americans sees their doctor every year because of cough. It stands to reason that there are many people just like Bob who have had to endure countless doctor visits without symptom relief, leaving them frustrated and discouraged. However, there is hope for chronic cough sufferers. Based on my years of experience in diagnosing and treating chronic cough, coupled with a thorough understanding of the science on this subject, I have developed a systematic approach to figuring out the source of chronic cough (see Figure 4).

THE FIRST STEPS IN FIGURING OUT YOUR COUGH

All investigations of chronic cough should start with eliminating smoking. That means cigarettes, cigars, and marijuana all have to go. For those who think pot smoking is for some reason okay, consider this: Smoking a single joint is the equivalent of smoking an entire pack of cigarettes.

Cigar smokers who believe that not inhaling cigar smoke leaves them immune from any carcinogens are deathly wrong. After escorting countless cigar-smoking, "I never inhale" patients into the operating room to remove part of their tongue, lip, or cheek, I can't stress enough the destructive carcinogenic effects of tobacco, regardless of how it is wrapped.

Once smoking is out of the picture, the next step is to see your primary care doctor. There, any infectious source of your cough can be ruled out with blood testing and throat cultures. A lung source of your cough

Figure 4 The Dr. Aviv Cough Algorithm

A Method for the Efficient Diagnosis of Cough

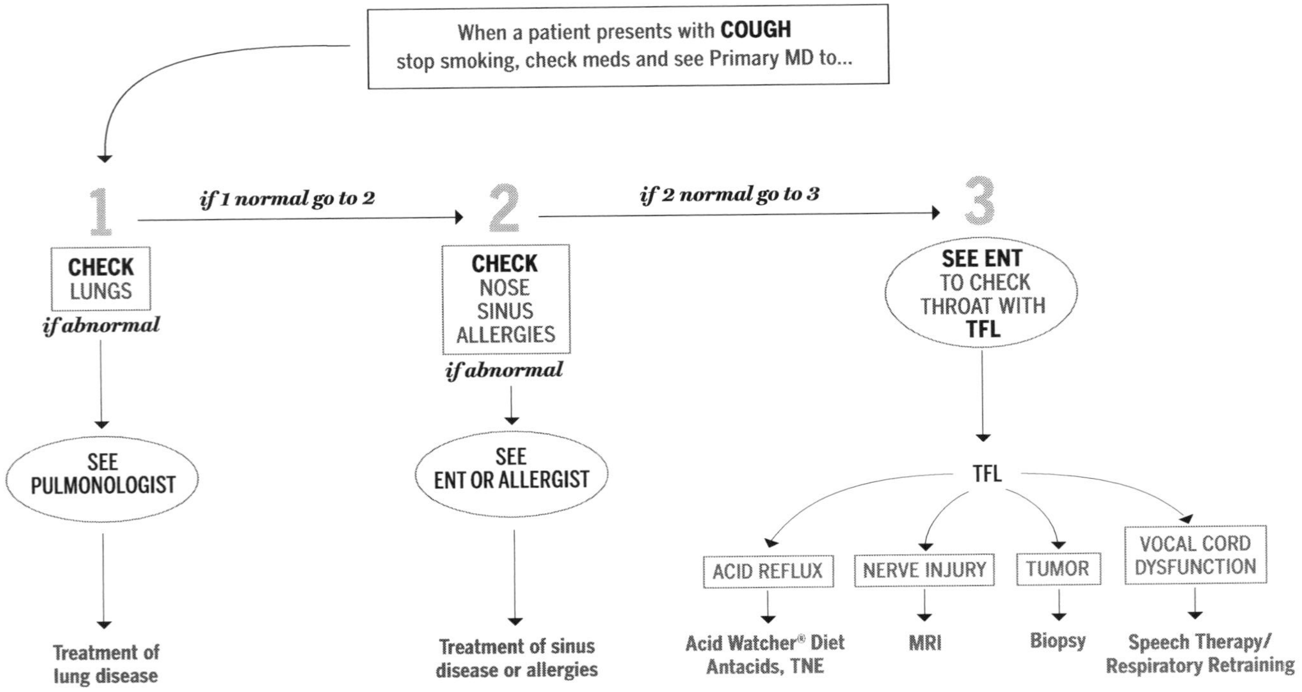

When a patient presents with **COUGH** stop smoking, check meds and see Primary MD to....

if 1 normal go to 2

if 2 normal go to 3

1

CHECK LUNGS

if abnormal

SEE PULMONOLOGIST

Treatment of lung disease

2

CHECK NOSE SINUS ALLERGIES

if abnormal

SEE ENT OR ALLERGIST

Treatment of sinus disease or allergies

3

SEE ENT TO CHECK THROAT WITH **TFL**

TFL

ACID REFLUX

Acid Watcher® Diet Antacids, TNE

NERVE INJURY

MRI

TUMOR

Biopsy

VOCAL CORD DYSFUNCTION

Speech Therapy/ Respiratory Retraining

Figure 4 The Dr. Aviv Cough Algorithm (previous page). When you have a chronic cough, the first thing you should do is stop smoking. Next, check your medications, as some can cause cough. Then, problems with the lungs, allergies, nose, and sinuses should be ruled out as the source. If ruled out, turn attention to your throat, where an Ear, Nose & Throat (ENT) physician performs an examination of the throat using Transnasal Flexible Laryngoscopy (TFL). The most common cause of unexplained cough is acid reflux, specifically Throatburn Reflux (or LPR). If signs of acid reflux are seen, a low-acid diet such as the Acid Watcher® Diet and medical treatment are used. Also, a TransNasal Esophagoscopy (TNE) should be considered to make sure no pre-cancerous conditions exist in the esophagus. After acid reflux is contemplated and ruled out, you must then consider nerve injury, tumor, or vocal cord dysfunction as the source of the cough. If a nerve injury such as vocal fold paralysis is seen, then imaging such as a Magnetic Resonance Imaging (MRI) of the neck is performed to make sure there is no tumor pressing on the nerve in the neck that moves the vocal fold. If a tumor is seen on the vocal fold during the exam of the throat, then a biopsy of the tumor should take place. Finally, if vocal cord dysfunction is seen, then appropriate treatment should commence (see Appendix B).

is then investigated, starting with your doctor listening to your chest to make sure your breath sounds are equal and clear. If your physician hears something abnormal, then further examination with a chest X-ray may be ordered to check for pneumonia, bronchitis, or lung cancer. A review of your medications is made to ensure that a class of blood pressure medicines called Angiotensin-Converting Enzyme (ACE) inhibitors are not being taken since chronic cough is a common side effect of this type of medication. ACE inhibitors have generic names that end with the four letters "pril"—for example, capto**pril**, mono**pril**, enalo**pril**. *Please do not suddenly stop your blood pressure medications*! Rather, speak with your doctor to determine a possible alternative medicine.

If the source of your cough has still not been determined, often a therapeutic trial of asthma medicines is implemented. If that doesn't provide relief, a pulmonary (lung) specialist consult should be obtained to formally diagnose asthma or other lung diseases as the cause of your cough. Sometimes, a computerized tomography (CT) scan of your chest may be ordered.

If the chest/lung evaluation is non-contributory, then allergies and paranasal sinus disease should be considered and a course of nasal steroid sprays, antihistamines, and decongestants should be tried. If unsuccessful, you should be referred to an allergist to determine if food or environmental allergens are the cause. With persistent symptoms, the final stop on the cough journey is to an ENT doctor such as myself. People with chronic cough are almost never referred to a GI doctor.

The Dr. Aviv Cough Algorithm is intended to give you an easy-to-follow guide to what otherwise would be a long, arduous process in determining the root cause of your chronic cough. As a doctor, I always worry about the things I can't see. For example, I can't see the lungs and I can't see subtle food and environmental allergens. So when a patient comes to me with chronic cough and they have already stopped smoking, have a normal chest X-ray, no ACE-inhibitors on board, and have been cleared by their lung doctor, I can then focus on the things I *can* see. I can see the throat. I can see the vocal folds. I can see the esophagus. Once seen, I am then able to help the patient start their recovery.

WHEN COUGH MASKS ACID REFLUX DISEASE

Chronic cough from acid reflux disease is epidemic, but pinpointing acid injury as the cause of chronic cough can be elusive. Take the case of my patient, Alice, a 34-year-old teacher who came to my office complaining of chronic cough that she had been suffering from for almost 10 years.

Like most of my patients, Alice had been thoroughly evaluated by numerous doctors for years, including internists, allergists, pulmonologists, and infectious disease specialists. Her chest X-ray and blood tests were normal. An extensive allergy investigation revealed no environmental or food allergies. Testing for asthma was negative. Even more sophisticated testing was performed such as CT scans of her paranasal sinuses and chest, also negative.

Four years prior to seeing me, Alice was prescribed antacid medications, which she took for three weeks without relief, so she stopped taking them. Alice mentioned that she didn't understand why she was given antacid pills in the first place since she didn't have any heartburn. *Starting to see a recurring theme*?

Once Alice's history was obtained, I examined her and began to unravel the source of her cough.

ENDING THE ENDLESS SAGA: THE CORRECT DIAGNOSIS

The first exam I performed on Alice was known as Transnasal Flexible Laryngoscopy (TFL). The prefix "trans" mean "through", so *transnasal* means through the nose. The use of the word *laryngoscopy* indicates that the larynx is being examined. The purpose of going through the nose to examine the larynx is mainly to bypass the strong gag reflex most of us have that exists in the back of the mouth. The miniature TFL camera is embedded at the tip of an instrument that not only looks as thin as a cooked piece of spaghetti, but is just as soft and flexible.

I sprayed a little numbing medication into Alice's nose and, a few minutes later, inserted the TFL instrument into her nose to get to her throat, which lies in the back of her nose. Once in that region, I was able to look at Alice's vocal folds and surrounding tissues. The camera was connected to a television monitor that displayed Alice's vocal folds. This allowed me to digitally record the exam for later review with Alice and to keep a visual record of her exam for future comparison.

I believe that when a patient can visualize what's going on in their own body, as they can with video-TFL, it's a great method of helping patients understand the impact of their lifestyle and eating habits on their internal organs. To see me performing a TFL on *The Dr. Oz Show*, please visit the following URL: http://www.entandallergy.com/vas/media.php ("What Your Voice Is Telling You").

DIAGNOSIS AND TREATMENT

In Alice's case, I found no evidence of any cancer or pre-cancerous conditions. There were no vocal fold movement problems, such as vocal fold paralysis. However, the test *did* show swelling of her vocal folds and the surrounding area near the opening of the esophagus. This was most likely the result of repeated and prolonged acid damage. I was then able to make my diagnosis—Throatburn Reflux.

I prescribed an appropriate treatment for Alice that included two distinct parts. The first included several dietary adjustments which will be reviewed shortly. The second involved Alice taking two classes of antacid medications—a proton pump inhibitor (PPI) (Table 4.1) in the morning and a Histamine-2 (H2) Blocker (Table 4.2) at bedtime. PPIs are the most powerful class of antacid medications. A single dose suppresses stomach acid for up to 16 hours. PPIs are finicky in that to be most effective they must be taken 30–60 minutes before eating. After taking a PPI, one must eat something within the 30–60 minute time frame (after taking the medication) in order to properly activate the medication. H2 Blockers, while highly effective, generally suppress acid for less than eight hours and, unlike PPIs, do not have to be taken before meals to be effective. I further explained to Alice that her cough would take about three months to improve.

Table 4.1
Common Proton Pump Inhibitors
(Brand name in parentheses)

Dexlansoprazole (Dexilant)

Esomeprazole (Nexium)

Lansoprazole (Prevacid)

Omeprazole (Prilosec)

Omeprazole/sodium carbonate (Zegerid)

Pantoprazole (Protonix)

Rabeprazole (Aciphex)

Table 4.2
Common Histamine-2 Receptor Antagonists (H2RA)
(Brand name in parentheses)

Famotidine (Pepcid)

Nizatidine (Axid)

Ranitidine (Zantac)

In general, only 25% of patients with Throatburn Reflux symptoms improve after six weeks of treatment with PPIs. Roughly 75% improve at 12 weeks, and 25% may require medication for six months or longer before they begin to feel better. This is why dietary and lifestyle changes are not only recommended, but absolutely necessary.

Although our society expects to have a "magic pill" to cure any ailment, the main part of Alice's treatment required discipline on her part. Specifically, she needed to make long-term dietary changes, understanding that even one highly acidic meal could bring her acid reflux symptoms back. In other words, medication alone is not enough.

Take-out Corner
Studies have shown that 80% of Americans are taking their Proton Pump Inhibitors (PPIs) incorrectly. The proper way to take a PPI is 30-60 minutes before you eat either breakfast or dinner, or both (allowing it to enter your blood stream). In addition, one must eat something to "activate" the PPI within 30-60 minutes after taking the medication.

POSITIVE RESULTS

Fortunately, Alice took what I told her to heart. When she returned for a follow-up exam three months after her initial diagnosis, the swelling in her larynx was vastly improved. She had completely cut out soda (one of her main food addictions) from her diet. She had also fully incorporated my low-acid, nutritionally balanced diet, called the Acid Watcher® Diet. (Chapter 8 describes my Acid Watcher® Diet and provides a detailed plan for breakfast, lunch, dinner, and snack options).

By following my recommended diet, an added benefit for Alice was losing nearly 15 pounds in those three months. In previous attempts at dieting, she had never been able to keep the weight off long-term. She told me that she found that she was a lot more motivated to commit to this new dietary change after actually seeing, via TFL, the damage a highly acidic diet had done to her throat.

SETTING EXPECTATIONS

It is essential that you understand that relief from the symptoms of Throatburn Reflux can sometimes take as long as three to six months. Too often, patients give up only a few weeks into their treatment because they don't see immediate results.

"But, Doctor," I've often heard patients say, "I tried that antacid medication, but it didn't work."

"How long did you use it for?" I would ask.

"Two weeks," is usually what I hear.

No one is going to see improvement in acid-related throat complaints with only two weeks of taking antacid medications. It takes a long time to reverse the changes of acid injury to the larynx.

Therefore, a great amount of discipline and commitment are required. Unfortunately, many patients fall off the wagon when it comes to both their medical and dietary regimens. Since most people ultimately don't want to have to depend on medications for the treatment of their acid reflux disease, diet will ultimately be the mainstay of their treatment.

SUMMING IT UP

It is important to remember that a chronic cough, regardless of what you have been told, is under no circumstances a normal health condition. I have provided you a road map to help you navigate your search for the proper health care and treatment you deserve.

The next chapter addresses one of the more dire possible consequences of untreated chronic cough—esophageal cancer.

5

ESOPHAGEAL CANCER PREVENTION: TARGETING THE RIGHT SYMPTOMS

*"When one door closes another opens. But often
we look so long and regretfully on the closed door we
fail to see the one that has opened for us."*

—HELEN KELLER

The unfortunate reality regarding esophageal cancer is that most people are at an advanced stage of the disease at the time they are diagnosed, with the survival rate usually being less than one year. The only way to make a dent in this disease is to catch it before it starts, while it is still in its pre-cancerous phase, called Barrett esophagus (see Chapter 3).

However, the current screening paradigm for esophageal cancer dictates that essentially only people who complain of heartburn should be examined for Barrett esophagus. Yet this approach is ineffective in preventing cancer since the majority of people with Barrett esophagus don't experience heartburn due to the numbness of the esophageal tissue caused by acid damage over the years.

Take-out Corner
The patients who are primarily at risk for esophageal cancer are not the ones being examined.

Think of the entire sequence of acid-induced injury as follows: Acid causes a burn. The burn then causes swelling of the tissues.

When tissues are swollen, sensitivity is diminished, leading to numbness.

In graphic form, this would appear as:

Acid → Burn → Swelling → Numbness

Over the past 10 years, research has shown that patients with throat symptoms, such as chronic cough, hoarseness, or a lump-like sensation in the throat, are the ones with the greatest risk of developing esophageal adenocarcinoma. Regrettably, these patients are not being examined for Barrett esophagus. This could, in part, explain why esophageal cancer is on the rise.

The time has come to change the way we think about acid reflux disease. This change involves understanding the connection between the stomach and the throat. Unfortunately, changing our habits and beliefs is much easier said than done, but this is precisely what it will take to connect the damaging impact of acid reflux disease with symptoms beyond heartburn.

"YOU WANT ME TO WASH MY HANDS?"

One of my favorite stories about how difficult it is to get new habits and beliefs accepted into the medical mainstream involves a hygienic practice which today is considered the standard of care, but was once thought of as not necessary. I'm referring to handwashing prior to performing surgery or any other medical procedure to prevent infection.

While this might be hard to believe, up until the late 1800s, all medical and surgical procedures were performed with bare hands, without handwashing or use of gloves. In the 1840s, a Hungarian-born doctor, Ignaz Semmelweis, who practiced obstetrics and

> **Take-out Corner**
> The majority of people with Barrett esophagus don't experience heartburn due to the numbness of their esophageal tissue caused by acid damage over the years.

gynecology in Vienna, noticed that mothers delivering babies in the section of his hospital that was staffed by medical students died at birth twice as often as in the ward staffed by midwives.

Upon investigation, Dr. Semmelweis found out that the students delivering babies with their bare hands had been previously working on cadavers at an adjacent facility. Although accepted germ theory had yet to be proven, Dr. Semmelweis believed that the medical students were transferring something from the cadavers on to the mothers, which caused them to become ill. Eventually, he was successful in getting the medical students to start washing their hands with a solution of chlorinated lime after handling cadavers. Subsequently, the mortality rate of mothers attended to by medical students at Semmelweis' hospital dropped by over 90%.

Unfortunately, when Dr. Semmelweis tried to get physicians outside his hospital to start washing their hands prior to performing medical procedures, he wasn't taken seriously and was, in fact, shunned by the medical community. The prevailing wisdom among doctors at that time was that handwashing was not only irrelevant, but also below their status and just too cumbersome.

Ultimately, Dr. Semmelweis' theory about handwashing proved too radical for its day and his efforts to change this were fruitless. Tragically, at the age of 47, he was committed to a mental institution where, within two weeks, he was severely beaten by the guards there and died from his injuries.

Fourteen years later, in 1879, at the Academy of Medicine in Paris, a physician was giving a lecture deriding the idea of handwashing.

Suddenly, in the middle of his speech, an audience member jumped out of his chair, passionately disagreeing with the expert lecturer. "The thing that kills women with childbirth fever," the man shouted, "is you doctors that carry deadly microbes from sick women to healthy ones!" This audience member was none other than Louis Pasteur, one of the founding fathers of the germ theory of disease.

It took over 50 years and countless lives lost for the idea of handwashing to be accepted from the time Dr. Semmelweis first suggested it. To this day, it's impossible to imagine patient care without handwashing. According to the Centers for Disease Control and Prevention (CDC), "Handwashing is the single most important means of preventing the spread of infection."

SCREENING VS. TARGETED INDIVIDUAL DIAGNOSTIC EFFORT (TIDE)

In today's complex medical world, changing the perception of which symptoms require further evaluation can be just as controversial as handwashing was back in the 19th century. The reasons can be ideological, financial, or practical, and may develop from a lack of skills, technology, or even knowledge.

The connection between Throatburn Reflux and esophageal cancer requires that patients with Throatburn symptoms have their esophagus examined. However, the idea of examining the esophagus in patients with throat symptoms has been misinterpreted by the anti-screening community as advocating widespread screening for esophageal cancer. This couldn't be further from the truth.

To be clear, I am not advocating the examination of healthy people who have no symptoms of the disease (the definition of screening).

I believe that one of the best solutions to halting the rapidly increasing incidence of esophageal cancer would be to implement a new strategy I call a *Targeted Individual Diagnostic Effort*, or TIDE. TIDE aligns current scientific data regarding acid reflux disease with how it should currently be diagnosed and treated.

TIDE will require educating the medical community, as well as patients, about acid reflux disease and its wide spectrum of symptoms beyond heartburn. As a result, TIDE will focus attention on throat symptoms, such as chronic cough, hoarseness, frequent throat clearing, and a lump-like sensation in the throat as *alarm symptoms* calling for the examination of the esophagus.

Focusing on the correct symptoms for an effective esophageal cancer prevention strategy is just part of the picture. What would make this pursuit even more efficient is the availability of a safe and inexpensive way to examine the esophagus. Fortunately, such a technique has been developed, although its potential hasn't been widely utilized yet. It is called TransNasal Esophagoscopy (TNE). TNE is a crucial piece of the puzzle that would allow TIDE to become an effective strategy in preventing esophageal cancer. To help you understand why TNE is different from any other esophageal examination technique available today, let's take a brief look at the history of esophageal examination.

THE HISTORY OF ESOPHAGEAL EXAMINATION

Examination of the esophagus began in the early 1900s through the efforts of the renowned American otolaryngologist, Dr. Chevalier Jackson, who pioneered rigid esophagoscopy. He inserted the instrument through the mouth of conscious patients who were lying flat on their back. The instrument was a two-foot long, hollow, stainless steel *rigid* rod, the width of an adult thumb, with a light at the tip. Don't try this at home.

Even today, rigid esophagoscopy remains the primary way to examine the esophagus in the ENT community. The main difference between the way Dr. Jackson performed this procedure and the way we do it now is the addition of general anesthesia for the patients. General anesthesia involves complete, deep sedation which includes placing a breathing tube into the lungs and putting the patient on a respirator for the duration of the procedure. Powerful sedating medications are typically required during general anesthesia. Though necessary for numerous procedures, general anesthesia has a series of known risks associated with it, including stroke, heart attack, heart rhythm problems, and drops in blood pressure.

Furthermore, even in highly trained hands, it is risky to pass a foot-and-a-half long, stiff rod into the esophagus. In addition, it is not that easy to see tissues at the far end of a thin cylinder. As a result, other medical specialists began to develop different esophageal examination techniques which proved not only safer, but much more comfortable for the patient.

The most popular of the alternative techniques to rigid esophagoscopy is *flexible* esophagoscopy, developed in the 1960s by the GI community. This procedure, which examines the esophagus, stomach, and upper part of the small intestine, is called Esophago-GastroDuodenoscopy (EGD, or upper GI endoscopy). During EGD, patients are placed in a twilight-type of anesthesia called **conscious sedation**. With

> ## ⧫ Take-out Corner
> Individuals complaining of chronic cough and hoarseness are at the greatest risk for esophageal cancer. The traditional esophageal cancer screening paradigms have been ineffective because they have targeted relatively lower-risk people such as those with heartburn.

conscious sedation, medicine is given into the vein to produce just enough sedation to keep the patient awake and breathing on their own, but "knocked out" enough so as not to feel discomfort or gagging.

However, conscious sedation EGD is not a panacea either, as any intravenous sedation has its risks. In fact, the most common cause of complications related to EGD is not from the procedure itself, but from the consequences of conscious sedation such as respiratory arrest (stopping breathing), stroke, and heart attack. While these instances are rare, there's no reason to undergo the risks of conscious sedation when an alternative procedure is available. This alternative procedure is TNE—the only technique that examines the esophagus without using sedation of any sort. By eliminating the risks of sedation, TNE can become the most effective diagnostic method in esophageal cancer prevention.

To appreciate the full impact of TNE, it's important to understand its development over the years.

NECESSITY IS THE MOTHER OF INVENTION: TRANSNASAL ESOPHAGOSCOPY (TNE)

Around the time I experienced my choking episode, there was almost no talk about the connection between esophageal cancer and throat symptoms. It was my personal experience with acid reflux and my invention of FEESST that pointed me toward the concept of acid causing so much damage in the throat that numbness of the throat structures could occur (as mentioned in Chapter 3). If I could readily see what was going on in the esophagus, it would add a more comprehensive dimension to determining the source of the throat complaints my patients were experiencing. The key, I felt, was getting into the esophagus without sedating the patient.

While researching various approaches to the esophagus in awake patients, I came across two scientific papers in the ENT and GI fields related to unsedated esophagoscopy. The first paper, published in 1993 by a South African pediatric otolaryngologist named C.A. Prescott, described a modified bronchoscope which was then passed into the esophagus. A bronchoscope is a thin, flexible camera that goes through the nose to examine the windpipe and lungs. While Prescott was essentially describing a transnasal esophagoscopy, his paper received little attention in the ENT world because its main focus was the examination of the esophagus in children after they swallowed caustic substances.

The second paper, published one year later by a GI physician in Milwaukee, Wisconsin named Reza Shaker, was the first paper to describe unsedated, transnasal EGD (T-EGD). Here, a thin, flexible camera was inserted via the awake patient's nose all the way through the esophagus, stomach, and first part of the small intestine.

Even though Dr. Shaker's work was a big step forward in the GI field, I couldn't use his exact technique since the T-EGD camera was too long and ENT doctors were not trained to look at the stomach and intestines. Nevertheless, Dr. Shaker's concept provided me the spark to the next step.

One day in November 1996, a month after my middle-of-the-night choking episode, I was speaking to Nicholas Tsaclas, one of the sales managers at Pentax Precision Instrument Corporation (Pentax). Pentax licensed the FEESST technology, so I had developed a close relationship with Pentax and Nick. Nick is one of the most knowledgeable medical device sales specialists in the country. During one of Nick's visits, he brought in a bronchoscope for me to look at.

While holding the bronchoscope, a thought occurred to me. Instead of

Take-out Corner◥

By placing the TNE camera through the nose, as opposed to through the mouth, one effectively bypasses the gag reflex which sits in the back of the mouth.

going into the lungs, the normal path when using a bronchoscope, what if I used it to look into the esophagus instead?

With Nick's agreement, I placed the flexible bronchoscope through his nose, then passed the scope all the way down to the bottom of his esophagus. Lo and behold, I was able to see that Nick had Barrett esophagus! At that moment, TNE was born. I now knew that, as an ENT doctor, I would be able to examine the esophagus without sedating patients, in an office setting, and without the risks that accompany general anesthesia and conscious sedation. Importantly, by placing the TNE camera through the nose, as opposed to through the mouth, I could effectively bypass the gag reflex which sits in the back of the mouth.

Fortunately for Nick, his Barrett esophagus has been followed successfully for years with serial TNEs and EGDs since that initial diagnosis, and his disease has not progressed. To see me performing a TNE on Nick on *Good Morning America*, please visit the following site: http://www.entandallergy.com/vas/media.php.

I continued to work on improving TNE technology by collaborating with several medical device companies (PENTAX, Medtronic, and Vision Sciences) to progressively shrink the width of the instrument. Today it has the diameter of a single strand of spaghetti. Further refinements of the TNE technology have included the development of a single-use disposable sheath (Vision Sciences) that slides over the camera to prevent cross-contamination when performing the procedure (see Figures 5.1, 5.2, 5.3). In addition, the sheath allows one to take biopsies of the esophagus by allowing a single-use, disposable biopsy tool (Medtronic) to be passed through a side channel embedded within the sheath (see Figures 5.4, 5.5, 5.6).

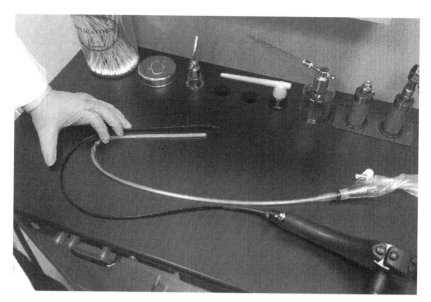

Figure 5.1 The TNE scope is lying next to next to the disposable TNE sheath. The sheath will slide over the scope to act as an infection barrier.

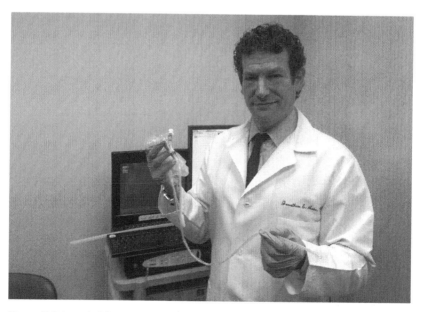

Figure 5.2 I am holding just the disposable sheath that covers the TNE scope. In my right hand, which is raised higher than my left hand, is the portion of the sheath that covers the handle of the scope. In my left hand is the part of the sheath that covers the tip of the scope.

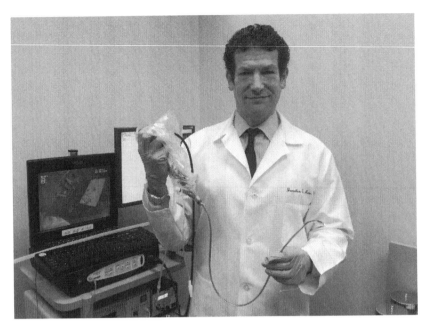

Figure 5.3 I am now holding the TNE scope with the TNE sheath placed over the scope. My right hand, raised higher than the left, is holding the scope handle, and my left hand is holding the tip of the sheathed scope.

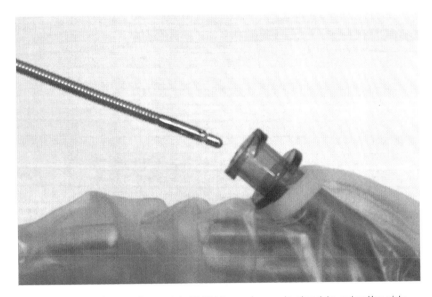

Figure 5.4 A single-use disposable TNE biopsy forcep is about to enter the side channel of the TNE sheath. Note that the biopsy forcep is in a closed position.

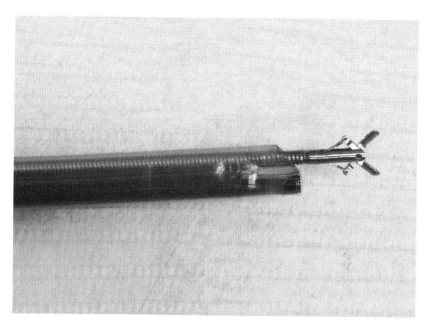

Figure 5.5 The single-use, disposable TNE biopsy instrument is shown coming out of the tip of the TNE biopsy sheath. The biopsy instrument is now open.

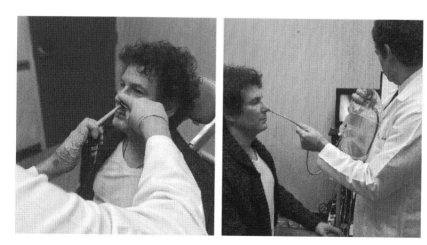

Figure 5.6 Patient receiving a TNE. *Left photo:* Patient's nose being sprayed with numbing medicine prior to the TNE procedure. *Right photo:* The TNE camera is passed through the nose into the esophagus. I am looking to my right at a television monitor which gives me a real time image coming from the TNE scope. This allows me to precisely examine the anatomy of the esophagus as well as the entire throat area.

GETTING CLOSER

Finally, in 2000, at the Combined Otolaryngologic Spring Meetings (COSM) conference in Orlando, Florida, I presented the findings on my first 14 TNE cases to a sparse audience.

Surprisingly, when I submitted the paper I presented at the conference for peer-review, it was initially rejected. Gratefully, the ENT Chairman at Columbia University at the time, Dr. Lanny Close, never wavered in his support of this new technique. I'll never forget what he said. "Jonathan, don't worry at all about this rejection. This is very important work and another journal will be happy to publish it."

Dr. Close was right, and in 2001 the official journal of the American Academy of Otolaryngology–Head and Neck Surgery published my first paper on TNE.

Several other key investigators in the ENT community, notably Drs. Jamie Koufman, Peter Belafsky, Greg Postma, Milan Amin, Gaelyn Garrett, and Michael Setzen, almost immediately began performing TNE. They have published extensively about their various applications of this technique in identifying LPR (Throatburn Reflux) patients at risk for esophageal cancer.

Over the past 13 years I have performed TNE in over 1,500 patients. I detected Barrett esophagus in approximately 15% of those patients, all of whom had Throatburn Reflux symptoms, *none of whom had heartburn.*

Take-out Corner

Because no intravenous medication is required for sedation during TNE, it becomes much safer for patients. Monitoring of the patient's heart rate, blood pressure, or oxygen levels is not required and there is minimal recovery time necessary.

ACCEPTANCE AND CHANGE

TNE is the state-of-the-art medical procedure performed on wide-awake patients to examine their esophagus for any pre-cancerous lesions. TNE does not require intravenous sedation, but it does require a small dose of numbing and decongestant medicine misted into the nose.

The procedure is so safe and lacking discomfort that I've performed TNE several times on national TV, including *ABC's Good Morning America, The Dr. Oz Show,* and *Bloomberg Television.*

TNE is more than simply inserting a tiny, flexible camera into the esophagus. The physician performing a TNE is also examining the inside of the nose and sinuses to make sure there is no significant sinus or allergy disease on the way down through the pharynx into the larynx. While in the pharynx, I make sure there are no tumors on the tongue and throat. A key portion of the procedure is to then examine the vocal fold area for signs of Throatburn Reflux disease. I next enter the esophagus and examine it entirely, including the bottom portion of the esophagus and the top portion of the stomach. In many cases, biopsies of the esophagus are performed during TNE.

It is important to reiterate that when no intravenous medication is required for any medical procedure, including TNE, the procedure becomes much safer. Monitoring of the patient's heart rate, blood pressure, or oxygen levels is not required, and there is minimal recovery time. Patients can instantly resume what they were doing before the exam.

IMPLEMENTING TNE

Unfortunately, Throatburn Reflux has flown under the radar of most GI doctors as well as ENT doctors and has resulted in TNE not being implemented to its full potential. From the mid-1990s to early 2000s, I was one of only a handful of physicians around the country performing

> ### ▶ Take-out Corner
> As of the publication of this book, over the past 13 years that I have been routinely performing TNE, over 1,500 cases, I have detected Barrett esophagus in about 15% of patients with chronic cough who had no heartburn.

TNE. Over the past 10 years, TNE has grown more common, but it is still only practiced by a few voice and swallowing sub-specialist ENT doctors called laryngologists, and even fewer GI doctors in this country.

Fortunately, as the data about the seriousness of Throatburn Reflux has become more convincing, the ENT community has started to implement TNE in residency training programs. In this way, the next generation of ENT doctors will not only know about the issue of Throatburn Reflux, but will be able to spot the deleterious effects of acid reflux disease using TNE.

The issue with GI doctors is completely different. One of the main impediments to the widespread adoption of TNE by the GI physician community is that they may be uncomfortable passing an instrument through the nose. The nasal cavity is an area of anatomy not thoroughly addressed in GI residency programs. However, this is a hurdle that can be overcome with post-graduate training courses, as almost all physicians are required to take continuing education courses. Therefore, hands-on instruction regarding the anatomy of the nose as it relates to TNE would be a natural path towards incorporating this procedure into their practices.

A more significant impediment to the shift to non-sedated esophagoscopy in the GI world may be that the facilities that perform sedated upper endoscopy receive a "facility fee" from insurance companies, including the U.S. government (Medicare, Medicaid), of about $1,000 per procedure. The facility fee covers the greater amount of monitoring, equipment, and personnel required to carry out sedation procedures. At roughly 10 million sedated EGDs performed each year, the cumulative cost approaches $10 billion annually. This is a major source of revenue for facility managers around the country, most

Take-out Corner
The fact that Throatburn Reflux has unfortunately flown under the radar of most GI doctors and even ENT doctors has resulted in TNE not being implemented to its full potential.

of whom would be unlikely to switch to a form of the exam that doesn't require sedation.

It is estimated that 50% of all EGDs are performed solely because of esophageal complaints. Studies have shown that in the absence of abdominal pain and nausea, TNE can effectively replace EGD for the examination of the esophagus. This would be a lot safer for the patient and more cost effective. The conversion from conscious sedation EGD to non-sedation TNE could potentially save the healthcare industry at least **$5 billion a year**.

I believe TNE will eventually play a pivotal role in the prevention of esophageal cancer. In the meantime, the following two things need to happen. First, patients with persistent cough, hoarseness, throat clearing, and globus sensation, as part of a TIDE (Targeted Individual Diagnostic Effort), *should have their esophagus examined.* Second, the decision to perform a sedated endoscopy (EGD) should be tempered by a technique that is safer for patients (TNE).

TNE: MYTHS AND FACTS

MYTH #1: TNE is not as well tolerated as conventional endoscopy (EGD).

FACT: From 1996 until now, there have been numerous studies comparing TNE and EGD, demonstrating that patients can tolerate a camera in their nose as well as they tolerate a camera in their mouth.

MYTH #2: TNE is not as effective as EGD.

FACT: Unsedated TNE has demonstrated equal accuracy in the detection of Barrett esophagus when compared with conventional, sedated, transoral upper endoscopy.

MYTH #3: TNE is expensive.

FACT: TNE is one-fifth the cost of EGD.

MYTH #4: TNE will increase our national healthcare costs.

FACT: TNE can save the healthcare industry about $5 billion per year.

MYTH #5: TNE has side effects.

FACT: Beyond the potential for a nosebleed, TNE is exceedingly safe.

EMPOWERING YOU

You have the ability to choose between an unhealthy, *burning body* as detailed in the first section of this book, and a *healthy body* which is described in the next section. I will take you through a step-by-step process to understand the logic and science behind selecting the best foods and healthiest lifestyle possible. This will give you the greatest opportunity to be as acid-free as possible. Consequently, you will thrive and improve your overall well-being.

PART 2
THE HEALTHY BODY

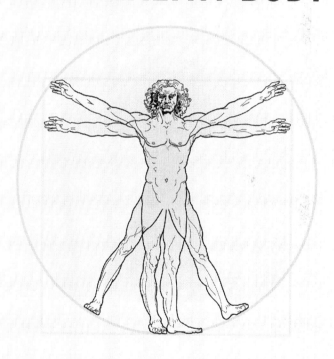

6

THE BUILDING BLOCKS OF THE ACID WATCHER® DIET:
How Carbohydrates, Proteins, and Fats Affect Our Bodies

"Tell me what you eat, and I will tell you what you are."
—JEAN ANTHELME BRILLAT-SAVARIN

The foundation for a healthy body starts with the Acid Watcher® Diet. It is a diet that I developed over the past several years which can help you transform your burning, highly acidic body into a healthy, balanced one. Its primary function is to help treat acid reflux disease and aid in preventing its complications, including Barrett esophagus and esophageal cancer. This diet was developed as a result of over 20 years of treating patients with these conditions.

In addition, a pleasant by-product of this diet is weight loss in patients who need it. In a sense, the philosophy of the Acid Watcher® Diet is almost in complete contrast to the way most other diets are presented. Most common diets say, "Lose weight first, then you will reap the health benefits." The fact is, losing weight is not a guarantee that you will be healthier. I have numerous patients who exercise regularly, are slim and trim, and appear to be extremely healthy, but still suffer from acid reflux disease. This was not because they couldn't diet or watch their food intake. In fact, their discipline with their regular food regimen was exemplary. Rather, their problem was that without even knowing it, they were eat-

ing the wrong types of food which exacerbated their acid reflux disease.

In contrast to this common way of dieting, the Acid Watcher® Diet is based on a very different type of philosophy—become healthy first and weight loss will follow. The main goal is a healthy and balanced body, not only a skinny body. With this in mind, my diet relies upon three crucial components:

1. Low-acid foods
2. A balance of healthy macronutrients
3. A high concentration of fiber

Before we get into the diet and meal plans, let's try and first understand how these three important factors affect our bodies and how they are applied in The Acid Watcher® Diet. I would like to start with macronutrients as this is the basis upon which the other two components are layered.

MACRONUTRIENTS

Food consists of three macronutrients—carbohydrates (including fiber), protein, and fat. Each macronutrient has a purpose in maintaining a healthy body. Macronutrients also contain micronutrients such as vitamins and minerals.

Many popular diets are often based on depriving your body of one macronutrient or another, such as a "low-fat" diet or a "low-carb" diet. Yet, that is why these diets are often unsustainable and sometimes even unhealthy. In contrast, the Acid Watcher® Diet offers optimal amounts of all three macronutrients, preventing any vitamin deficiency, loss of energy, sugar or salt cravings, and numerous health issues that can arise as a result of following an unbalanced diet.

Besides vitamins and minerals, macronutrients contain compounds called **phytochemicals** that boast profound health benefits such as reducing inflammation and preventing certain cancers. To better understand what phytochemicals are, think of them as substances that give plants their color, taste, smell, and texture. Some familiar examples would be carotenoids that give vegetables their red-orange color, such as in carrots and sweet potatoes, or isothiocyanates that give kale and broccoli their earthy flavor.

Unfortunately, the industrialization of our food supply since the 1970s, which I talked about in the previous part of the book, has impacted our ability to get these nutrients to the table. For example, pesticides used in farming can inhibit plant-based foods from developing natural phytochemicals. That is why you've probably noticed that non-organic vegetables don't have as strong a scent, flavor, and color as organically grown vegetables. Furthermore, during food processing and preserving, micronutrients are often drastically reduced or bleached out of the food, such as in "white" bread or "white" rice. In addition, how one cooks plant-based foods can affect their nutritional value as well. That's why the Acid Watcher® Diet avoids processed foods but does include plenty of organic raw fruits and vegetables, as well as steamed veggies.

Take-out Corner
The lists of ingredients printed on the packaging of processed foods are becoming ever longer, containing words we can't pronounce whose meaning we don't understand.

I stress the importance of a nutritionally balanced way of eating because the mass industrialization of our natural food supply has made it very difficult for people to balance their intake of macronutrients. This is primarily because it's often hard, even for a doctor like myself, to know or understand what our food is actually made of. The lists of ingredients printed on the packaging of processed foods contain ever longer words we can't pronounce and whose meaning we don't understand.

The following sections detail what sources of macronutrients you should eat, what to avoid, and what impact they have on acid reflux disease.

CARBOHYDRATES—WHY WE NEED THEM

Many diets that try to regulate the intake of carbohydrates have come and gone. But one thing we know for sure—carbs remain an essential source of energy for your brain, muscles, and heart. Based on their molecular complexity, carbohydrates are divided into two groups: complex carbs and simple carbs.

Complex (Good) Carbs

Complex carbohydrates are broken down into sugar gradually over a longer period of time than simple carbs due to their more complex molecular structure. This allows for a slow, gradual release of sugar into the bloodstream, providing the body with a steady, more balanced source of energy. After consuming complex carbs, blood sugar levels should remain relatively stable. Table 6.1 gives examples of natural sources of complex carbs.

Table 6.1
Natural Sources of Common Complex (Good) Carbohydrates
*These foods are highly acidic and should be avoided for those with acid reflux disease

Vegetables	Whole grains	Legumes
Broccoli	Brown rice	Beans (all types)
Cucumber	Oats	
Cauliflower	Whole grain cereal	**Fruit**
Spinach	Whole wheat pasta	Apricots
Lettuce (all types)	Whole wheat bread	Apple
Potatoes	Whole grain bread	Pear
Corn		Prunes
Carrots	**Dairy**	Plum*
	Milk	Orange*
	Cheese	Grapefruit*
	Yogurt	

Simple (Bad) Carbs

As its name suggests, simple carbs have a much simpler molecular structure than complex carbs. For that reason, they get broken down into sugar very rapidly, often causing drastic sugar spikes in the blood.

Unfortunately, simple carbs form the foundation of most processed or commercially baked goods, such as cookies, doughnuts, chocolate, potato chips, soda, as well as thousands of other packaged foods we eat daily. In fact, almost all pre-packaged foods, juices, sweeteners, "low-fat" food, "low-cal" food, and most food made with white flour, such as white pasta and white bread, contain simple carbs (see Table 6.2).

When one consumes an excessive amount of simple carbs, especially from processed and refined foods devoid of fiber, instead of fueling the body with energy, it will actually leave one feeling deprived. For example, eating a large piece of chocolate cake on an empty stomach will result in an immediate burst of energy, but a couple of hours later, fatigue will set in. What actually happens when an excessive amount of sugar rapidly reaches the blood

> **Take-out Corner**
> Simple carbs, as the name suggests, have a much simpler molecular structure than complex carbs. As a result, they get broken down into glucose very rapidly, often causing drastic sugar spikes in the blood.

is that the pancreas starts producing large amounts of insulin until the blood sugar level drops. Once the blood sugar level drops, one often starts feeling tired, which can lead to a craving for even more sugar. That is why one will then often reach for the ice cream sitting in the freezer, and the process starts all over again.

This is dangerous because unchecked sugar cravings over time predispose a person, not only to acid reflux disease, but to obesity, diabetes, heart disease, and other physical maladies that plague so many of us living on a "Western" diet.

Table 6.2
Simple Carbs That Should Be Avoided

Fruit juices
Soft drinks
Table sugar
Cakes
Cookies (packaged or otherwise)
Candy
White bread
White pasta
Ice cream
Anything that contains high fructose corn syrup

It's important to note that many fruits and vegetables contain naturally occurring simple carbs, but that doesn't mean they should be avoided, since they often contain fiber and a wide variety of vitamins and minerals that your body needs. However, I would proceed with caution when it comes to fruit juices, even naturally squeezed, as they contain very little or no fiber. Therefore, the sugar in those juices reaches your blood stream a lot faster, causing an unhealthy sugar spike.

FIBER: AN ACID REFLUXER'S FRIEND

A good rule of thumb, whether you suffer from acid reflux disease or not, is that you should always eat a diet rich in fiber. According to the American Heart Association, the average American consumes around 15 grams of fiber a day. This is way too low for consistent healthy digestion. You should be eating 25–35 grams a day, something recommended by the Academy of Nutrition and Dietetics. Although there are many fiber supplements on the market today, it is much better for acid reflux sufferers, as well as everyone else, to get their fiber from natural foods. In addition to the actual fiber, natural foods contain vitamins and minerals that aid in the alkalization, or buffering, of our stomach acid.

Fiber can be defined as that part of food, whether from a fruit, vegetable, nut, bean, or grain, that can't be broken down or digested to be turned into body energy. Fiber itself contains no calories, which is why foods with a high proportion of fiber (broccoli, spinach, celery, and kale) are very low in calories. In addition, foods high in fiber make you feel satiated with smaller food volumes. As a result, foods rich in fiber can be very helpful in weight loss. Pointedly, animal products do not contain fiber.

The reason that the Acid Watcher® Diet emphasizes consumption of adequate amounts of fiber is that it acts in a mechanical and chemical way to prevent acid reflux. Mechanically, fiber aids digestion by helping the body get rid of waste and toxins from our intestines. It acts much like a wide, stiff-bristled broom, sweeping through our intestines and colon, keeping it clean. This can alleviate pressure on the lower esophageal sphincter (LES, see Chapter 2). Fiber also works chemically, regulating blood sugar levels by slowing down the conversion of carbohydrates into

---

Take-out Corner

Whether you suffer from acid reflux disease or not, your carbs should come from foods rich in fiber.

sugar (glucose), thereby eliminating cravings. Since one of the main causes of acid
reflux is overeating, increasing natural fiber
in one's diet is a great way to stop stuffing
yourself.

Table 6.3 lists a variety of popular foods
that are rich in fiber that are excellent for acid reflux disease sufferers.
Though berries have a lot of fiber, they are also acidic. However, as you'll
soon see in Chapter 8, their acidity can be neutralized or lessened by mixing them with other more alkaline foods.

Table 6.3
High-Fiber Foods

Vegetables	**Grains**	**Nuts/Seeds**
Broccoli	Brown rice	Almonds
Brussels sprouts	Oat & wheat bran	Walnuts
Asparagus	Whole grain cereals	Flax seed
Potatoes	Whole grain breads	Sunflower
Beets	Buckwheat	Pecans
Carrots	Barley	
Cucumbers	Rye	**Legumes/Beans**
Seaweed		Lentils
All green leafy veggies	**Fruit**	Chick peas
	Apples	Lima beans
	Berries	Peas
	Banana	
	Avocados	
	Pears	

PROTEINS—WHY WE NEED THEM

Protein is a crucial macronutrient that helps our body grow and repair
itself. This is particularly important for most acid reflux patients who
have an inflamed or damaged esophagus, since protein can help repair
affected tissue.

Protein is also a main component of our cells and organs. Every cell in
the body contains some form of protein. Muscles are almost completely
made up of different proteins. The same is true for our hair, skin, and eyes.

Take-out Corner
Some sources of protein are very high in saturated fat, such as red meat. This can affect the ability of the Lower Esophageal Sphincter (LES) to function properly.

Many other important chemicals in our body, such as hormones and enzymes, which help regulate digestion, are also made up of protein.

As you may have surmised by now, anything that can help with digestion is a crucial component in the diet of an acid reflux disease sufferer. In the case of protein, it's not just a question of having enough protein, but the *type* of protein as well (see Table 6.4).

When you choose your protein source, it's very important to consider the overall nutritional value of that particular type of food. Some sources of protein are very high in saturated fat, such as red meat. Excessive amounts of fat can exacerbate acid reflux by impairing the ability of the LES to function optimally. This can lead to stomach acid flowing unimpeded up and out of the stomach, where it can injure the esophagus. (For a refresher on this concept, please refer back to Chapter 2.)

Table 6.4
Examples of Good Protein Sources for Acid Reflux Sufferers

Animal Sources of Healthy Protein	Vegetable Sources of Healthy Protein
Sardines	Peanuts
Salmon	Oatmeal
Tuna	Beans (all types)
Halibut	Cashews
Turkey—light meat, no skin	Almonds
Chicken—light meat, no skin	Tofu
Yogurt	Edamame
Kefir	Walnuts
Eggs	Soy milk
	(non-genetically modified organism (GMO))
	Hazelnuts
	Whole grains
	Quinoa
	Broccoli
	Spinach
	Kale
	Spirulina

Beans and eggs, especially egg yolks, can be hard for some people to digest. I recommend that they be consumed in moderation. Animal sources of protein should primarily be eaten in combination with vegetables (fiber) for easier digestion, especially when the consumed vegetables are either raw or steamed.

FATS—WHY WE NEED THEM

Fat is one of the most crucial components of the human body. A healthy body is made up of 20% fat, with our brain being made up of 60% fat. Fat helps regulate our body temperature and protects our internal organs from impact injury. It is also important for maintaining healthy levels of hormone production and joint lubrication. In addition, fat helps keep our nerve structure in place, which is crucial for neural transmission. Many essential vitamins and minerals only get absorbed by our bodies if they are attached to fat.

Therefore, the Acid Watcher® Diet focuses on replacing *bad* fats with *good* fats, and there's a huge difference between the two. Let's get the bad out of the way first.

Trans Fats *(bad fats)*

Trans fat should absolutely be avoided by anyone with acid reflux disease. In fact, trans fat should be avoided by everyone. Most trans fats that make it onto our plates are formed during the processing of food in order to turn fat into a solid, as well as to make our processed food last longer. Ever wonder why that box of crackers you bought during the Clinton Administration is still so crispy and fresh? Thank you, trans fat.

Trans fat is formed when hydrogen ions are blasted into vegetable oil under pressure to make the fat more stiff. As a result, trans fat also goes under the catch-all name "hydrogenated oil." Margarine, cookies, potato chips, microwave popcorn, and most "healthy" butter-like substances are examples

> ▶ **Take-out Corner**
> Trans fats shouldn't just be avoided solely by acid reflux sufferers. They should be avoided by everyone.

of trans fat in a pretty package.

Trans fat is bad for several reasons. It increases low-density lipoprotein (LDL or "bad cholesterol") levels, while at the same time decreasing high-density lipoprotein (HDL or "good cholesterol") levels. This significantly increases our risk for heart disease. In addition, for acid reflux sufferers, trans fat loosens the LES so stomach acid can freely splash back up into the esophagus (see Chapter 2).

Now, for the good news on fat.

Unsaturated Fats (good fats)

MONOUNSATURATED FATS

Monounsaturated fats are considered to be a good type of fat when consumed in moderation. They help increase our body's HDL levels while lowering our body's LDL. These fats are liquid at room temperature but will solidify when refrigerated. They're found in a wide variety of foods, such as meat, whole milk, olives and olive oil, avocados, almonds, cashews, and peanuts. With the exception of red meat, monounsaturated fats are typically good choices for people with acid reflux disease (see Table 6.5).

However, there is a subset of monounsaturated fat that is not good for those with acid reflux, such as vegetable oils made from seeds. Examples include soybean oil, corn oil, canola oil, safflower oil, cottonseed oil, grape seed oil, and sunflower oil. These seed oils usually require high-tech processing using extreme heat, pressure, and/or chemical solvents in order for the oil to be extracted. High heat destabilizes the molecular structure of these oils, resulting in free radical formation which is highly inflammatory and caustic to the body.

"Cold-pressed" vegetable oils are always the best option to use for an acid reflux sufferer. If possible, choose extra virgin olive oil, which is oil that was extracted from the first pressing of the olive fruit. Additional pressings produce oil of a lesser quality. If you've ever had a chance to smell and taste homemade olive oil, you know that it has a very distinct and strong scent. Olive oil without a scent has probably been heavily processed or deodorized and should be avoided.

Table 6.5
Common Monounsaturated Fats of Choice for Acid Reflux Sufferers:

Cold-pressed extra virgin olive oil
Avocado and avocado oil
Cashews
Almonds
Peanuts

POLYUNSATURATED FATS (OMEGA-3 & OMEGA-6)

Polyunsaturated fat is one of the healthiest forms of fat. Two of the more important subcategories of polyunsaturated fat are omega-3 and omega-6 fats. They are considered "essential" fat because they cannot be produced by our bodies and must be obtained through the consumption of food (see Table 6.6).

Omega-3 is produced in the leafy parts of the plant during photosynthesis. Omega-6 is produced predominantly in the seeds of plants. Animals acquire the largest amount of omega-3 fats by directly consuming leafy plants or grass. That is why meat or eggs from grass-fed animals will have more omega-3 than grain-fed animals.

Fish is also a very potent source of omega-3 fat. Fish acquire their omega-3 from eating algae or plankton naturally found in the ocean. However, not all fish are created equal. Just like with land animals allowed to run free and eat grass for their

> ▌**Take-out Corner**
> Oils that are made from seeds (such as cottonseed and grape seed oil) require special processing with extreme heat, pressure, and often chemical solvents in order for the oil to be extracted. Extreme heat changes the molecular structure and nutritional value of oil, making it less healthy.

sustenance, wild fish are richer in omega-3 than farmed fish. In addition, cold-water fish has the highest amount of omega-3 because their natural habitat promotes the best conditions for the accumulation of this type of fat in their bodies.

Omega-3 is considered to be one of the most beneficial types of fat as it helps maintain the integrity and the permeability of our cell walls. It also helps metabolize glucose (sugar), lowers cholesterol, and supports brain function.

Omega-6 fatty acids are found in seeds, grains, nuts, and vegetable oils such as canola and sunflower oil. Even though certain types of omega-6 fats have undeniable health benefits, the Western diet is, to say the least, excessive in omega-6 consumption, mainly due to the high intake of processed food, which is rich in seed oils.

Table 6.6
Common Polyunsaturated Fats

Omega-3 rich food	Omega-6 rich food
Salmon	Seed oils (canola, sunflower, grapeseed)
Anchovies	Sunflower seeds
Herring	Pumpkin seeds
Mackerel	Poultry
Trout	Eggs
Sardines	Avocado
Halibut	Pecans
Tuna	Cashews
Eggs (from grass-fed chickens)	
Spinach	
Kale	
Seaweed	
Flaxseed	
Walnuts	
Marine algae	

Much research has been done trying to find the ideal ratio between omega-6 and omega-3 consumption. However, I believe that it is very difficult for anyone who is not a scientist to fully understand what these numbers really mean in a practical sense. Therefore, I would like to simplify this issue to the following take-home message—remove processed and deep-fried food from your diet. At the same time, increase your fish intake to at least twice a week and eat plenty of vegetables so your body will find a natural balance between omega-6 and omega-3 fat.

SATURATED FATS

Saturated fat can be found in both animals and vegetables. The fatty layer under your skin that regulates your body temperature consists of saturated fat. However, the plaque in your arteries is also made up of saturated fat.

What usually makes saturated fat harmful to our health is not just the processing it often undergoes before reaching our dinner tables, but the sheer amount of it that we eat. Since saturated fat usually makes up the majority of our daily diet, it shouldn't surprise you that a highly saturated fat diet is often a major contributor to acid reflux disease.

It's important to note that the "processing" of our food starts way before the food has been packaged, boxed, and shipped to the local supermarket. Animals raised on most feedlots in the U.S. typically spend their lives being fed excessive amounts of grains, antibiotics, and growth hormones. Hardly ever do they see direct sunlight during their short lives. This is one of the reasons why I recommend that whenever you eat eggs, dairy, or meat, it should ideally be organic and come from a grass-fed animal.

If you don't have access to organic animal products, try to replace them with fat found in plants (avocado, coconut, olives, nuts, seeds), or the healthy fat found in fish, as discussed in the previous section. Although saturated fat is needed in our bodies, excessive amounts are harmful. One of the most important points to remember regarding our food

> **Take-out Corner**
> By removing processed and deep-fried food from your diet and increasing your fish intake to at least twice a week, along with eating plenty of vegetables, you should find a natural balance between omega-6 and omega-3 fats.

Take-out Corner

One of the most important points to remember regarding our food intake is that moderation does not mean "midway," as in 50/50. In the case of saturated fat, if you really want a percentage-type guide to follow, do not have more than 10% of your daily fat intake come from saturated fat food.

intake is that moderation does not mean "midway," as in 50/50. In the case of saturated fat, if you really want a percentage-type guide to follow, do not allow more than 10% of your daily fat intake to come from saturated fat.

"Fat-Free"? "Low-Fat"? Puh-lease!

It seems that the ongoing crusade to promote and consume low-fat items has failed to make us a healthy and skinny nation. Perhaps with our best intentions, we continue to mistake "fat-free" or "low-fat" items for healthy. It should be obvious by now that this is simply not the case.

I was recently shopping for some plain yogurt and got distracted by the colorful labels on the fruit yogurts. All the available types, and there were plenty of them, were either "fat-free" or "low-fat." I couldn't find a regular fruit yogurt anywhere. Now, you might be thinking, "What's wrong with that?" What's wrong is the flawed logic to think that by simply removing or decreasing one macronutrient from our diets, we can ultimately improve our overall health.

Take-out Corner

"As I scanned the label of one of the yogurts that is highly praised and popular for its numerous health claims, I realized that the sugar content was 23 grams per 113 grams of yogurt. That's the equivalent of eating almost five teaspoons of pure sugar in one sitting—just as a snack!"

Nature is a lot more complex than that. As I scanned the label of one of the fruit yogurts that is both highly praised and popular for its numerous health claims, I realized that its sugar content was 23 grams per 113 grams of yogurt. That's the equivalent of eating almost five teaspoons of pure sugar in one sitting— just as a snack! It's even more preposterous when you consider that yogurt is supposed to be one of nature's healthy foods.

At first, one might think that the yogurt, labeled "fat-free," couldn't be that bad. After all, the fat was presumably removed from the yogurt. However, that's actually where the problem lies. Fat gives us a sense of

▼ Take-out Corner

Regardless of a person's dietary goals, carbohydrates, proteins, and fats are essential to a well-balanced diet.

satiation, or the sense of feeling full. But with fat-free food, we tend to eat a lot more. In a sense, we chase that sense of fullness, while inadvertently ingesting excessive (and even harmful) amounts of sugar along the way.

In addition, another important property of fat is that it creates flavor. Without fat, food manufacturers often have to add a lot of sugar and/or artificial flavors to make their food tasty. Our overall national health will not improve by demonizing and expelling macronutrients from our food. Our health will only improve when we stop adding unnecessary artificial components to our food.

MACRONUTRIENT SUMMARY

In the end, there's no escaping the fact that carbohydrates, proteins, and fats are essential to our health. There are many dietary trends that come and go, just like shoes, cars, clothing, and hairstyles. But please try not to fall for them. Always aim for balance with your eating choices and habits.

Before we begin to look at the Acid Watcher® Diet as a well-balanced dietary program for reducing acid reflux, there is one last item that is important for you to understand. When a person suffers from acid reflux disease, there is one main litmus test—understanding pH and its effect on our bodies.

7

pH BASICS AND THE pH OF COMMONLY CONSUMED FOODS

"The wise man should consider that health is the greatest of human blessings. Let food be your medicine."
—HIPPOCRATES

You may recall from your high school chemistry class that every organic solution is either acidic or alkaline. This applies to any type of fluid, including fluids from food, as well as bodily fluids. The pH level is a measure of how acidic or alkaline a particular solution is. It refers to the concentration or density of hydrogen ions in that solution. The stronger the concentration of hydrogen ions, the more acidic the solution is.

Every substance below pH 7 is considered acidic, while everything above pH 7 is considered alkaline. Figure 7 provides a way to better visualize this important concept. This figure associates common substances with their corresponding pH value.

There are a lot of misconceptions about how the pH level of food affects the human body. Some of the misunderstanding comes from failing to take into account that pH levels in the body are dynamic and vary from organ to organ, depending on the function they perform. For example, the pH level of skin is around 5.5, which is slightly acidic, while the pH

Figure 7 Overview of pH Values of Common Substances

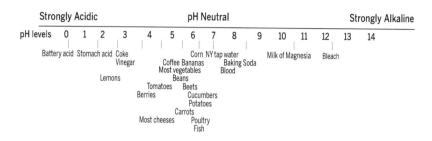

level of saliva is more on the alkaline side, ranging from 6.5–7.5. The pH level of blood falls within the narrow range of 7.35–7.45. Unfortunately, we often experience health problems when any of the aforementioned pH values fall out of their optimal range.

The pH levels throughout our body mostly depend upon what we ingest, as well as our lifestyle and habits. This includes what we eat or drink, if we smoke or take drugs, our daily stress level, as well as our exercise and sleeping habits.

WHY ACID REFLUXERS SHOULD BE WARY OF THE ALKALINE ASH DIET

In most cases, acid reflux disease can be prevented by maintaining a proper diet. However, my patients are often confused about what to eat and what not to eat. On a daily basis, my patients ask me questions like, "Should I drink apple cider vinegar for my reflux? I heard it's a natural cure," or, "Is it true that lemon juice can heal heartburn?"

I believe that most of these questions are a result of the popular alkaline ash diet and other similar diets that claim that food, after being digested, leaves either an acidic or alkaline residue in the body. For exam-

◤Take-out Corner

Every part of the body has its own ideal pH level. The normal pH level of stomach acid is between 1.0–4.0. Saliva is more alkaline, while our skin is more acidic. When these levels fall out of their optimal range, our health can become compromised.

ple, it's said that lemon leaves an "alkaline residue" and therefore it's good for the alkalization of the body. However, as it relates to acid reflux, the alkaline ash theory is not applicable because it fails to take into consideration the possibility that food itself can cause damage to the throat and esophagus. This occurs because of the possibility of **pepsin** being present in the throat and esophagus.

Pepsin is an enzyme released by the stomach whose primary function is to break down protein. Pepsin has two forms: Inactive and active. In its inactive form, pepsin is basically "asleep" in the stomach. Pepsin only gets activated or "woken up" when exposed to acid, at which point it starts breaking down the protein in the food that is present in the stomach after a meal.

However, if even a small amount of stomach acid reaches the throat, pepsin molecules will travel along with it and become attached to the throat and esophagus like Velcro. The pepsin can then stay in the throat for an extremely long period of time, going in and out of its "sleep mode." Every time you drink that lemon juice, soda, or apple cider vinegar, pepsin will "awaken" and can start eating away at the lining of your esophagus and/or severely inflame your vocal folds. The only way this process will stop is if there is no acid present in that area to keep the pepsin active.

Pepsin is most active in an environment that has a pH level between 1-4, and becomes progressively more *inactive* at pH 5 or greater. An acid reflux sufferer has to be very careful because pepsin is re-activated every time it encounters food that has a low pH level.

Now you can begin to understand why the alkaline ash diet is not a good choice for people who suffer from acid reflux. It ignores how the pH of ingested food affects the pepsin that already exists in the throat and esophagus. It would be similar to pouring acid over a wound. A very bad idea.

THE pH OF COMMONLY CONSUMED FOODS

The following series of tables provides the pH of commonly consumed foods and beverages, all of which were tested using a professional pH meter. The tables are separated into various food categories such as vegetables, fruits, roots, and dairy.

All acid reflux sufferers should ideally eat foods above pH 5. Another important point to keep in mind is that "green is good." Almost any vegetable, *especially the green ones*, are alkaline and very healthy for you.

Please keep in mind that there are a few exceptions to the above pH 5 "rule":

1. Garlic, onions, and peppers, while they are above pH 5, are also *carminatives*, which are a class of foods that loosen the LES and therefore should be avoided (see Chapter 2 for more information regarding the LES).

2. Canned beans, even though above pH 5 as well, often contain chemicals and preservatives, so fresh whole beans should be the first choice. If cooking fresh beans is not an option, then choose an organic brand of canned beans.

Table 7.1
pH of Commonly Consumed Raw Vegetables

Cucumber (English)	**7.6**	**Kale**	**6.01**
Zucchini	**6.8**	**Cabbage**	**5.98**
Cauliflower	**6.72**	**Lettuce (Arugula)**	**5.92**
Lettuce (Romaine)	**6.6**	**Basil**	**5.92**
Spinach	**6.5**	**Parsley (fresh)**	**5.65**
Broccoli	**6.28**	**Cucumber (Garden)**	**5.44**
Celery	**6.24**	***Orange pepper**	**5.2**
Lettuce (Iceberg)	**6.23**	***Green bell pepper**	**5.2**
Swiss chard (raw)	**6.22**	*Yellow bell pepper	4.8
Asparagus (raw)	**6.21**	*Red bell pepper	4.8
Cilantro (fresh)	**6.18**	Grape tomato	4.5

Table 7.2
pH of Commonly Consumed Raw Fruits

Avocado	**7.12**	Apple (Gala)	4.31
Black Olives		Prunes (dried)	4.27
(Cerignola, in water)	**7.10**	Peach (yellow, ripe)	4.25
Watermelon	**6.53**	Pear (Forelle, ripe)	4.20
Cantaloupe	**6.42**	Blueberries	4.19
Lychee	**5.91**	Pear (Bartlett, ripe)	4.15
Butternut Squash (raw)	**5.81**	Grapes (green seedless)	4.12
Banana	**5.71**	*Orange (Valencia)*	*3.89*
Papaya	**5.66**	*Strawberries*	*3.87*
Dates (Halawi, Delilah)	**5.49**	*Pineapple*	*3.87*
Dragon Fruit	**5.45**	*Apple (Honeycrisp)*	*3.79*
Honeydew	**5.42**	*Apple (Pink Lady)*	*3.75*
Pumpkin	**5.40**	*Orange (Mandarin)*	*3.75*
Pear (Bosc)	**5.15**	*Yellow grapefruit*	*3.74*
Apple (Red Delicious)	4.88	*Blackberries*	*3.74*
Kiwi	4.84	*Raspberries*	*3.56*
Mango	4.58	*Apple (green)*	*3.54*
Figs	4.55	*Plum*	*3.39*
Apple (Golden Delicious)	4.50	*Pomegranate*	*3.32*
Cherries	4.43	*Lime*	*2.55*
Raisins (dark)	4.41	*Lemon*	*2.45*

Table 7.3
pH of Commonly Consumed Roots

Mushrooms (Cremini)	6.79		Potato (Idaho, cooked)	5.95
Potato (red skin, cooked)	6.40		Sweet potato (cooked)	5.91
Ginger	6.28		Carrots (cooked)	5.83
Leeks	6.21		Beets (cooked)	5.79
Beets (raw)	6.19		*Onion (white, raw)	5.74
Carrot (raw)	6.14		*Onion (red, raw)	5.60
*Garlic	6.17		*Radish (red)	5.50
*Onion (sweet)	6.15		*Horseradish (raw)	5.35

Table 7.4
pH of Commonly Consumed Dairy Products

Blue cheese	6.99		Cottage cheese	4.64
Milk (fat free, Parmalat)	6.97		Butter (unsalted)	4.63
Whole milk (organic, Kirkland)	6.86		Feta cheese	4.60
Milk (grass fed, unhomogenized)	6.76		Cream cheese (Philadelphia)	4.59
Butter (salted)	5.86		Yogurt (plain, Stonefield)	4.43
Hard cheese (Dublin)	5.80		Greek yogurt (plain, Fage)	4.34
Hard cheese (Parmesan)	5.40		Goat cheese	4.32
Hard cheese (Asiago)	5.20		Greek yogurt (plain, Chobani)	4.31
Soft cheese (Mozzarella)	5.20		Kefir	4.17
Hard cheese (Cheddar)	5.16			

Table 7.5
pH of Eggs

Egg white	8.84
Egg (hard boiled, organic)	7.48
Egg yolk	6.32

Table 7.6
pH of Commonly Consumed Tree Nuts

Almonds (raw)	6.08
Walnuts (raw)	5.96
Cashews (salted)	5.41
Pistachios (salted)	5.33

Table 7.7
pH of Commonly Consumed Dairy Alternatives

Almond milk (vanilla, Silk)	8.40	Coconut milk, cultured (vanilla, So Delicious)	4.66
Almond milk (original flavor, Silk)	8.36	Soy yogurt (plain, Whole Soy & Co.)	4.64
Soy milk (plain)	7.94	Coconut milk, cultured (plain, So Delicious)	4.58
Tofu	6.90		
Rice milk (plain, organic)	6.35	Soy yogurt (vanilla, Whole Soy & Co.)	4.44
Almond yogurt (plain, Almond Dream)	4.67		

Table 7.8
pH of Commonly Consumed Condiments and Spreads

Almond butter (natural)	6.32	Mustard (Grey Poupon)	3.86
Peanut butter (fresh ground)	6.15	Ketchup	3.70
Bragg Liquid Aminos (soy sauce alternative)	5.00	Mustard (spicy brown, Gulden's)	3.68
Humus	4.37	Strawberry preserves	3.49
Agave	4.34	Cherry preserves	3.09
Honey (Manukah)	4.31	Raspberry preserves	3.06
Agave (light)	4.20	Apple cider vinegar	3.05
Mayonnaise	3.86	Balsamic vinegar	2.95

Table 7.9
pH of Commonly Consumed Waters

Evamor	8.80	NYC tap water (filtered- Multipure)	6.59
Aquadeco	7.78	Perrier	5.64
Jana	7.78	Dasani water	5.46
Glacéau smartwater	7.70	Coconut water (Zico)	5.26
Fuji	7.55	Distilled water	5.22
Evian	7.36	Hint water (strawberry)	3.80
Arizona Vapor Water	7.30	Vitamin water (grape)	2.93
NYC tap water (unfiltered)	7.23	Vitamin water (raspberry)	2.90
Voss flat water	6.68		

Table 7.10
pH of Commonly Consumed Beverages

Orange juice (Tropicana)	3.87	Cranberry juice (Ocean Spray)	2.56
Diet Coke	3.21	Coke	2.50
Diet Pepsi	3.04	Pepsi	2.46
Iced tea (peach, Snapple)	3.02		

Table 7.11
pH of Commonly Consumed Meats, Fish, and Seafood

Lobster (boiled)	7.30	Turkey (fresh, roasted)	6.17
Shrimp (boiled)	6.92	Sardines (fresh)	6.15
Crab meat	6.75	Tuna (seared)	6.10
Halibut (poached)	6.62	Cod (broiled)	6.05
Salmon (grilled)	6.32	Hamburger	5.80
Octopus (grilled)	6.30	Chicken (grilled)	5.23
Tuna (in water, canned)	6.18	Beef (sirloin)	5.10

Table 7.12
pH of Commonly Consumed Breads

Multigrain bread (Bread Alone)	5.53
Ezekiel 4:9 Flax	5.48
100% Whole grain bread	5.35
Ezekiel 4:9 Sesame	5.27
Whole wheat fiber bread	5.07
Ezekiel 4:9 Cinnamon Raisin	4.64

Table 7.13
pH of Commonly Consumed Legumes

Peas (green)	6.80
Peas (black-eyed)	6.62
Edamame	6.57
Cannellini (canned, organic)	6.10
Beans (canned, garbanzo, Goya)	6.04
Beans (canned, black, Goya)	5.93
Beans (canned, red, Goya)	5.87

Table 7.14
pH of Several Miscellaneous Foods

Liquid chlorophyll supplement (World Organic)	8.40
Wheat grass juice (fresh)	6.03
Pedialyte (unflavored, Abbot)	5.54
Carrots (baby food, jar, organic, Earth's Best)	5.02
Banana (baby food, jar, Earth's Best)	4.30
Pear (baby food, jar, Beach-Nut)	3.84
Apple and Cherry (baby food, organic, Happy Baby)	3.66

As you can see from the tables above, there are many food items that we eat which are very healthy, yet acidic, so they are not recommended for people suffering from acid reflux disease. An example of this is berries, which have an acidic pH of 3.34-4.19. Because berries are very nutritious, it's hard to recommend restricting them, especially as most people today consume fewer and fewer raw fruits. In the case of berries, however, I found that by blending them with certain high-alkaline foods, such as almond milk, soy milk, or rice milk, via a smoothie (the "Dr. Aviv Smoothie," whose recipe is found in Chapter 8), their acidity is lessened and brought to a safe pH level for people with acid reflux.

Now, let's take a look at the Acid Watcher® Diet. Before starting the diet, however, please consult your personal physician if you are taking any type of medication, are pregnant, or have any type of chronic disease.

With that said, it's time to turn the page towards a healthier you.

8

DR. AVIV'S ACID WATCHER® DIET: A DIET YOU CAN LIVE BY

"The doctor of the future will no longer treat the human frame with drugs, but rather will cure and prevent disease with nutrition."

—THOMAS EDISON

INTRODUCTION

The previous two chapters set the foundation for the Dr. Aviv Diet®, also known as the Acid Watcher® Diet. This is not only a new diet for you, but a lifestyle change as well.

Most modern diets that promise to help you shed pounds quickly are unsustainable. In addition, the typical popular diet is often not properly balanced with the macronutrients that your body needs. These diets are usually either a no-fat or a no-carb diet, or some version of a starvation diet. Healthy eating, as found in the Acid Watcher® Diet, is about balance and moderation. It is never about the complete exclusion of carbs, fat, or protein, but it *is* about the exclusion of highly acidic and processed foods.

> **Take-out Corner**
> Healthy eating, as found in the Acid Watcher® Diet, is about balance and moderation. It is never about the complete exclusion of carbs, fat, or protein.

The Acid Watcher® Diet consists of two parts: The **Healing Phase,** which lasts for the first four weeks of the Diet, followed by the **Sustainable Phase**, which is the diet that you should maintain to stay healthy and acid reflux free for the rest of your life.

PHASE 1 OF THE ACID WATCHER® DIET: THE HEALING PHASE

The Acid Watcher® Diet four-week Healing Phase is the period of time in which your body will begin to heal itself from years of acid damage. These initial four weeks are usually the hardest part of the Diet for everyone, since you have to restrict all meals to foods above pH 5. On the other hand, I've had numerous patients say that this was the most rewarding part of the Diet as they felt the greatest positive change in their bodies during this period of time.

The first step in starting the Healing Phase is to eliminate the main foods, substances, or habits that contribute to acid reflux disease, which I refer to as the "**non-negotiables**". There is a set of non-negotiable rules both for the Healing Phase as well as for the Sustainable Phase of the Acid Watcher® Diet.

As the term suggests, there is "no negotiation" when it comes to eliminating these harmful items in order to achieve success with the Diet. These are rules that you must follow.

The Acid Watcher® Diet Healing Phase "Non-Negotiables"

During the Healing Phase of the Diet (first four weeks of the Diet), there can be absolutely:

1. **NO** foods less than pH 5
2. **NO** alcohol
3. **NO** lying down within three hours after eating
4. **NO** carbonated beverages (including all sugary sodas, club soda, or sparkling water)
5. **NO** caffeine
6. **NO** prepackaged (processed) foods
7. **NO** deep-fried food
8. **NO** chocolate
9. **NO** food with mint (including gum)
10. **NO** smoking of any substance

Trigger Foods

If *any* of the foods you consume, regardless of their pH level, cause a negative reaction—either traditional Heartburn Reflux symptoms (heartburn or regurgitation) or Throatburn Reflux symptoms (chronic cough, hoarseness, constant throat clearing, or a lump-like sensation in the throat)—it's important to isolate, identify, and avoid that particular type of food.

Surprisingly, it is quite common to have one patient tolerate one type of food very well, only to find that another patient can't tolerate the identical food at all. Over the years, I've found that some common examples of these *trigger* foods are grapefruit, pineapple, tomato, coffee, caffeinated tea, alcohol, chocolate, onion, garlic, cow's milk, bread, and pasta. It is important to note that trigger foods can be almost anything, *regardless of their pH value.*

> **▼ Take-out Corner**
> Trigger foods can be almost anything, regardless of their pH value.

The Acid Watcher® Diet: *Must-Eat Foods*

Besides the "non-negotiables" which must be eliminated for the Acid Watcher® Diet to be effective, there is another aspect of the Diet which is equally important—the two *must-consume foods*. These need to be eaten on a daily basis to get the most out of the Acid Watcher® Diet.

Vegetables. Eat a daily minimum of one pound of vegetables, above pH 5, half of which should be raw. For example, five medium-size carrots is approximately a pound. Four handfuls of string beans is also approximately a pound, and five cups of spinach is about half a pound.

Fruit. Eat a daily minimum of a half a pound of raw fruit, above pH 5. For example, a handful of cubed cantaloupe with a banana is approximately half a pound. The fruit in a Dr. Aviv Smoothie (see below in the Recipe part of the chapter) is also roughly half a pound.

Since these two requirements are crucial to the success of the Acid Watcher® Diet, you should strive to reach these goals *daily*. Remember, that's a minimum of one pound of vegetables and a half a pound of fruit *every day*.

As far as choosing and combining different vegetables and fruits, you have the freedom to choose any variety above pH 5 during the Healing Phase, and any types above pH 4 during the Sustainable Phase of the Diet. It is important that you keep referring back to the pH tables from Chapter 7 until the values of all the foods that you consume become routine for you.

Meal Preparation Rules for Both Phases of the Acid Watcher® Diet

1. Foods that can't be eaten raw should either be grilled, steamed, poached, broiled, baked, or sautéed. This means no *deep-frying*.

2. I'd prefer that you use Celtic salt for seasoning as it is rich in minerals and not processed like most regular "white" salt is.

3. Salad dressing should consist only of fresh, cold-pressed virgin olive oil or coconut oil, with mineral Celtic salt. Alternatively, you can follow recipes for dressings found in the Acid Watcher® Diet.

4. If you are in a restaurant and want chicken or fish, order it steamed or grilled, without any sauce on it.

5. Your bread of choice should be 100% whole grain. Whole grain means that 100% of the original kernel of the grain (all of the bran, germ, and endosperm) must be present. This includes any whole grain such as rye, spelt, wheat, barley, and oat. When the grain has been broken into pieces as part of the bread-making process, all the parts must be utilized. Some examples are Bread Alone-Organic Whole Spelt Bread and Food For Life-Ezekiel 4:9 Bread Original Sprouted Organic. If you can't find 100% whole grain bread, then please choose a type of bread that doesn't have preservatives or artificial flavors.

6. Try and keep the use of oil down to a minimum, and always make sure the olive oil you use is of good quality and fresh.

7. If you eat poultry or fish for lunch, your dinner should be vegetarian. Conversely, a vegetarian lunch should be followed by a poultry or fish dinner.

8. If at all possible, please choose organic fruits and vegetables, especially when there is no protective covering such as a banana peel or watermelon shell.

Eat On Time

Both phases of the Acid Watcher® Diet provide a relatively strict eating program that incorporates five meals per day using the following time schedule:

7:00 AM–9:00 AM	Breakfast
10:00 AM–11:00 AM	Mid-morning Mini-Meal
12:30 PM–2:00 PM	Lunch
3:00 PM–4:00 PM	Mid-afternoon Mini-Meal
6:00 PM–7:30 PM	Dinner (kitchen closes at 7:30 PM)

It is crucial that you don't miss meals and that you eat within the suggested time frame. This helps avoid drops and spikes in blood sugar levels.

Liquids

The only beverage that should be consumed during the first month Healing Phase is water. For those who can't stand just water, one can add a cube of watermelon to make the water slightly sweeter. Alternatively, one can add a few thin slices of cucumber to make the water more savory.

Take-out Corner

It is crucial that you don't miss meals and that you eat your meals within the suggested time frame. This helps avoid drops or spikes in blood sugar levels.

BECOMING AN ACID WATCHER®

The Acid Watcher® Diet Healing Phase: MEAL PLAN

In order to make the Diet as easy to follow as possible, I've created a detailed weekly meal plan along with its corresponding shopping list and recipes. This weekly meal plan is to be repeated four consecutive times to complete your one month of healing (see Figure 8.1).

The recipes are created according to all the Acid Watcher* tenets that I've described in the book, requiring a relatively short amount of time for preparation. The meals are designed in such a way that even someone who doesn't have a lot of experience in the kitchen would be able to prepare them. Since most people work during the day, I also took into consideration that they don't have time for long meal preparation at lunchtime. That is why most lunches in the Diet can be eaten cold and be prepared the night before to be brought to work.

However, for those who have more time or are skillful in the kitchen, I've added some additional recipes that can occasionally be alternated with the recipes from the original Healing Phase meal plan, as long as the meals match according to the appropriate food categories. For example, an animal protein (AP) dish can be substituted for another AP dish, and a vegetarian (V) dish can be substituted for another V dish.

Figure 8.1
Acid Watcher® Diet: Weekly Healing Phase Meal Plan
(Repeated for 4 consecutive weeks)

	SUNDAY	MONDAY	TUESDAY	WEDNESDAY	THURSDAY	FRIDAY	SATURDAY
BREAKFAST 7–9 AM	F Dr. Aviv Smoothie	ED Spinach Omelet	G Banana Oatmeal	F Dr. Aviv Smoothie	ED Broccoli Omelet	G Pear Oatmeal	V Green Juice
MORNING MINI-MEAL 10–11 AM	V Guac Tapenade Toast	F Fresh Fruit 8 oz.	V Raw Veggies	ED Hard Boiled Egg	F Fresh Fruit 8 oz.	ED Mozzarella Herb Toast	N Toast with Almond Butter & Honey
LUNCH 12–2:30 PM	AP Dr. Aviv's Healthy Chicken Nuggets & Asparagus	V High Fiber Salad	AP Pesto Chicken Sandwich	V Kale Wrap	V Vegetable Pasta Salad	AP Colorful Chicken Salad	AP Broiled Salmon with Spinach
AFTERNOON MINI-MEAL 3–4 PM	NF Dr. Aviv Power Bar	N Assorted Tree Nuts	F Fresh Fruit 6–7 oz.	N Toast with Almond Butter	N Assorted Tree Nuts	F Fresh Fruit 5–6 oz.	F Fresh Fruit 8 oz.
DINNER 6–7:30 PM	V Kale Salad	AP Miso Halibut with Bok Choy	V Cream of Broccoli Soup, Sweet Potato	AP Turkey Burger with Arugula Salad	AP Fish & Chips	V Papaya Salad	V Roasted Vegetable Sandwich

AP =Animal Protein, ED =Eggs or Dairy, F =Fruit, G =Grain, N =Nut-based, NF =Nuts and Fruit, V =Vegetarian

The Acid Watcher® Diet Healing Phase: WEEKLY SHOPPING LIST

Below you will find your weekly shopping list for the Healing Phase of the Acid Watcher® Diet, which should be repeated for four consecutive weeks.

Please note that aside from proteins, fruits, and vegetables, almost all items purchased in the first week will carry over into the following weeks of the Diet. *To make this easy for you, I placed an asterisk next to each carryover item.* Please use organic fruits and vegetables when possible.

* = Food item that generally can be carried over beyond one week

Fish
5–6 oz. of salmon fillet (buy fresh for Saturday)
5–6 oz. of halibut fillet, skinless (buy fresh for Monday)
5–6 oz. Fresh fish fillet (tilapia, trout, flounder, branzino or sole—
    buy fresh for Thursday)

Poultry
1 lb. chicken breast
4–5 oz. ground turkey (buy fresh for Wednesday)

Eggs 12 eggs

Vegetables and Herbs
1 lb. spinach
1 head of Romaine lettuce
¼ lb. arugula
1 bunch of curly kale (for salad)
4–5 oz. (5–6 leaves) Lacinato kale (for juicing)
1–2 medium heads of bok choy
2 lbs. broccoli
1 bunch of asparagus
3 stalks of celery
2–3 cucumbers
1 small zucchini
1 small eggplant
1 yellow squash (non-GMO)
1 small potato
2 sweet potatoes
2 lbs. of carrots (don't use baby carrots)
1 raw beet

*1 stem of raw ginger

3–4 oz. green beans (fresh or frozen)

3–4 oz. of organic corn (fresh or frozen, non-GMO)

*1 small package of green peas (frozen)

3 oz. of Cremini mushrooms

*1 bunch of basil

*1 bunch of cilantro

*1 bunch of parsley

1 small package of fresh or dried rosemary

1 small package of fresh or dried herbs such as thyme/sage/savory

Olives
3 oz. of pitted Kalamata olives

Raw fruit
3–5 bananas

2 ripe Bosc pears

2 cups of mixed berries (blueberries, raspberries, blackberries, strawberries)

1 papaya (non-GMO)

2 ½ lbs. of your choice of fresh fruit: cantaloupe, watermelon, honeydew, ripe Bosc pear, banana, lychee

1–2 lemons

3 Hass avocados

Dried fruit
5 pitted Halawi dates

*1 small package of black raisins (without preservatives and coloring)

*1 small package of shredded coconut

Nuts and seeds (raw, unsalted)
*1 small package of pecans

2 oz. of your choice of either: cashews, pecans, pistachios

*1 small package of walnuts

*1 small package of pumpkin seeds (pepitas)

*1 small package of sesame seeds

*1 small package of almonds

*1 small package of pine nuts

Spreads
*1 small container of fresh, raw, organic peanut butter

*1 small container of fresh almond butter

Cheese
*½ lb. of crumbled feta cheese

*½ lb. of mozzarella cheese

4 oz. of grated parmesan cheese

Non-dairy milk
*½ gallon of non-dairy milk, either soy milk (non-GMO) or rice milk
*½ gallon of almond milk (unsweetened)

Bread/Grains
*1 small package of old fashioned rolled oats
*1 small package of whole grain fusilli pasta
 1 loaf of 100% whole grain bread
*1 small package of whole wheat flour

Sweeteners
*1 jar of honey (preferably raw honey)
*1 small jar of agave nectar

Additional Items/Condiments
*1 package of Celtic salt
*1 bottle of extra virgin olive oil or coconut oil
*1 bottle Bragg Liquid Aminos
*1 small package of hemp protein (optional for smoothies)
*1 small bottle of vanilla extract
*1 small container of white miso paste

The Acid Watcher® Diet Healing Phase: **RECIPES**

BREAKFAST 7:00–9:00 AM

Dr. Aviv Smoothie pH 5.96 | **F** | Serves 1

1 cup of blueberries or mixed berries

½ cup of almond milk

1 banana

3–4 ice cubes (optional)

Blend thoroughly and enjoy.

Notes: The almond milk neutralizes the acidity of the berries.

Modifications and additions: Add a handful of spinach to make **Dr. Aviv's Berry Smoothie Blast!** (pH 6.11).

Add 1 tablespoon of hemp protein to make **Dr. Aviv's Protein Smoothie** (pH 6.25).

MORNING Mini-Meal 10:00–11:00 AM

Guac Tapenade Toast pH 6.4 | **V** | Serves 1

6 Kalamata olives, pitted, drained of oil

½ Hass avocado

1 teaspoon of fresh cilantro, chopped

1 slice of toasted whole grain bread

Use a food processor to mash the olives, avocado, and cilantro, then spread on a slice of toasted bread.

Dr. Aviv's Healthy Chicken Nuggets and Asparagus

AP | Serves 1

4–5 oz. of boneless chicken breast

1 egg

2 tablespoons of whole wheat flour

½ teaspoon fresh rosemary, chopped

1 teaspoon fresh parsley, chopped

½ teaspoon of olive oil or coconut oil

Celtic salt to season

2–4 tablespoons of water

CHICKEN PREPARATION: Slice the chicken into thin 2" by 2" pieces. Season the chicken with salt and herbs. Cover with plastic wrap and pound down on the chicken, flip over, and pound the opposite side.

In a mixing bowl, beat the egg and add a pinch of salt. Dip the chicken into the egg, then place it in another bowl with flour and coat it on both sides. In a non-stick pan heat up the oil on medium and then place the chicken in it. Add 2–3 tablespoons of water to the pan. Cover and cook over medium heat. Flip the chicken over after 2–3 minutes. Keep the pan covered for a few more minutes or until all the water evaporates. The chicken is finished cooking once it turns a light brown color. Cooking time for the chicken should be approximately 5–6 minutes. If you like your chicken crispy, cook for an extra minute or two.

Asparagus

7–8 stalks of asparagus

1 teaspoon of olive oil or coconut oil

½ teaspoon of parmesan cheese for flavor (optional)

ASPARAGUS PREPARATION: Cut off the bottom ends of the asparagus. Heat up oil in a pan on low and add asparagus. Keep moving the asparagus in the pan until cooked so it won't stick to the pan and burn. After 2–3 minutes, add the parmesan cheese, stir into asparagus for a few seconds, and remove from pan. Be careful not to overcook the asparagus. The asparagus should stay crunchy.

AFTERNOON Mini-Meal 3:00–4:00 PM

Dr. Aviv Power Bar NF | Serves 1

5 pitted dates

20 almonds

1 tablespoon of organic, raw peanut butter

2 drops of vanilla extract

1 tablespoon of shredded coconut

In a food processor, add almonds and pitted dates. Grind well for a couple of minutes. Place this mixture into a small mixing bowl. Add the peanut butter and vanilla extract. Mix well with a spoon for a couple of minutes. Transfer the mixture to a cutting board, and shape it to resemble a standard "power" bar. Coat the bar with shredded coconut on both sides, and enjoy one of the healthiest power bars you'll ever eat!

DINNER 6:00–7:30 PM

Kale Salad V | Serves 1

1 large kale leaf (about 12 inches), chopped

3 teaspoons of finely chopped walnuts (make sure they are fresh!)

3 heaping tablespoons of freshly shredded carrots

⅓ of a cup of chopped cucumbers

½ teaspoon of fresh olive oil

10–15 raisins, cut into small pieces

5–6 Kalamata olives, chopped

2 tablespoons of crumbled feta cheese

Carrot-ginger dressing (see recipe below)

CARROT-GINGER DRESSING: pH 5.73 | V

4 tablespoons of raw carrots, shredded or chopped

1 tablespoon of olive oil

1 tablespoon of agave

¼ tablespoon of raw ginger, coarsely chopped

¼ teaspoon Celtic salt

¼ cup of water

CARROT-GINGER DRESSING PREP: Mix all the dressing ingredients in a food processor. Process it for about a minute, until you achieve a nice dressing-like consistency.

In a large bowl, mix all the salad ingredients together and add 3-4 tablespoons of the carrot-ginger dressing. Enjoy an incredibly healthy dinner!

MONDAY

BREAKFAST 7:00–9:00 AM

Spinach Omelet AP | Serves 1

1 whole egg

2 egg whites

½ teaspoon olive oil or coconut oil

1 tablespoon of green or black olives

1 teaspoon of grated parmesan cheese (optional)

Handful of raw spinach

1 slice of toasted whole grain bread

Chop up the olives. Heat up oil in a pan on low to medium heat. Add the eggs, olives, and cheese, and stir well. When the eggs are about halfway cooked, add the spinach and keep mixing. When the eggs are cooked through, turn off flame and serve.

Serve with 1 slice of toasted whole grain bread.

MORNING Mini-Meal 10:00–11:00 AM

Fresh Fruit 8 oz. F | Serves 1

8 oz. of fresh fruit

Choose from cantaloupe, papaya, watermelon, honeydew, ripe pear, banana, or lychee.

LUNCH 12:30–2:30 PM

High Fiber Salad 🥗 | Serves 1

2–3 oz. (3 large leaves) of Romaine lettuce, chopped

Handful of raw broccoli, chopped

½ cup of cucumber, chopped

3 tablespoons of carrots, shredded

5–6 pitted Kalamata olives, chopped

3 tablespoons of cooked green peas

3 tablespoons of raw beets, shredded

1 teaspoon of olive oil

2 tablespoons of crumbled feta cheese

Pinch of Celtic salt (optional)

1 slice of whole grain bread (optional)

Mix all the ingredients together. To prepare the green peas, either frozen or fresh, put in hot water, and bring to a boil. Drain the water and add them to your salad.

Modifications and additions: This recipe is flexible as long as all the vegetables you choose are above pH 5.

If you wish to cook the beets, cut them into 2-3 pieces, then place them in boiling water and cook until soft. Drain the water, let the beets cool off, slice them up, and add to your salad.

For the **Sustainable Phase** of the Diet (see page 122), you can add red or green bell peppers.

AFTERNOON Mini-Meal 3:00–4:00 PM

Assorted Tree Nuts 🥜 | Serves 1

1 oz. (about a handful) of your choice

Mix from walnuts, cashews, pecans, or pistachios.

Miso Agave Glazed Halibut with Sesame Bok Choy ⒶⓅ | Serves 1

5–6 oz. halibut fillet, boneless, skinless

1 tablespoon white miso paste

½ teaspoon agave

1–2 tablespoons water

1–2 medium heads of bok choy, roughly chopped

⅛ teaspoon Celtic salt

½ teaspoon olive oil

½ teaspoon sesame seeds

½ slice of toasted whole grain bread (optional)

In a medium size bowl, whisk together the miso, agave, and water. Place the halibut in the mixture and marinate for 15 minutes. Place on oiled aluminum foil, then put onto a baking pan and broil until golden brown and caramelized, about 5–7 minutes. Meanwhile, heat the ½ teaspoon of oil in a large sauté pan over medium heat. Add the bok choy and salt, and sauté until tender, about 1 minute. Sprinkle with sesame seeds.

Serve with ½ slice of toasted whole grain bread.

Modifications and additions: If you do not wish to glaze the fish, please refer to Saturday's lunch fish recipe.

BREAKFAST 7:00-9:00 AM

Banana Oatmeal with Pecans & Coconut Flakes ⑥ |

Serves 1

½ banana, cut up

½ cup non-dairy milk (soy milk (non-GMO), almond milk, or rice milk)

1 teaspoon honey

Pinch of Celtic salt

5 tablespoons of old fashioned rolled oats

1 tablespoon raw pecans, chopped

1 tablespoon coconut flakes

2-3 drops of vanilla extract (optional)

Cut half a banana into small pieces. In a saucepan, heat up the non-dairy milk and salt. Add oats and cook on medium heat, stirring constantly, until thick and creamy, about 2 minutes or so. Remove from the stove and add the banana, honey, pecans, coconut flakes, and vanilla extract. Mix well and serve.

MORNING Mini-Meal 10:00-11:00 AM

Raw Veggies Ⓥ | Serves 1

½ cup of raw veggies

Choose from carrots, celery, and cucumber. You can use a pinch of salt if necessary.

Pesto Chicken Sandwich 🔲 | Serves 1

4–5 oz. (about a palmful) of grilled or roasted chicken breast

2 teaspoons of pesto sauce

   (see recipes for dairy and non-dairy versions below)

2 thin slices of fresh buffalo mozzarella

2 leaves of romaine lettuce or a handful of arugula

2 medium slices of whole grain bread

1 teaspoon of olive oil

1 pinch of Celtic salt

CHICKEN PREP: Preheat oven to 450° F. Place the chicken in a roasting pan, sprinkle with olive oil and a pinch of salt, and place in the oven. Roast until cooked, about 10–15 minutes. Make sure you flip the chicken breast over about halfway through the roasting process. When the chicken is finished, let it cool off, then chop into small pieces.

PESTO SAUCE (NON-DAIRY) pH 5.38

2 cups of basil, packed

¼ cup of unsalted pine nuts

¼ cup of olive oil

PESTO SAUCE (DAIRY) pH 5.49

2 cups of basil, packed

¼ cup of unsalted pine nuts

¼ cup of olive oil

2 tablespoons parmesan cheese, grated

PESTO SAUCE PREP: Add all ingredients into food processor and mix until desired thickness is attained. Add a pinch of salt if necessary.

SANDWICH PREP: Add pesto sauce to the chicken and mix well. Place mozzarella and lettuce with the chicken in a sandwich and enjoy.

Modifications and additions: You can also use rotisserie chicken.

AFTERNOON Mini-Meal 3:00–4:00 PM

Fresh Fruit 6–7 oz. 🔳 | Serves 1

Choose one of the following options:

A) 1 cup of fresh fruit. Choose from cantaloupe, papaya, watermelon, honeydew or ripe Bosc pear.

B) 1 handful of peeled lychees with ½ cup of fruit listed above.

DINNER 6:00-7:30 PM

Cream of Broccoli Soup with Pepitas and Sweet Potato Fries dairy free | 🔳 | Serves 2

3 broccoli heads

2 teaspoons of Celtic salt

2 cups non-dairy milk (soy milk (non-GMO), almond milk, or rice milk)

½ Haas avocado

2 tablespoons of raw pepitas (pumpkin seeds)

1 teaspoon of olive oil (with a little more for seasoning)

SOUP PREP: Heat the olive oil in a large pot over a medium flame. Add the broccoli and salt. Sauté for about 5 minutes, then pour in the (non-dairy) milk. Bring to a boil, simmer until the broccoli becomes tender, about 5 more minutes.

Transfer half of the broccoli mixture to a blender, add the avocado, and blend until smooth and creamy. Pour into a bowl and add the rest of the broccoli mixture to the blender. Pulse a few times so that the broccoli is blended but still slightly chunky. Combine both broccoli mixes together. To serve, sprinkle with pepitas and drizzle with olive oil to taste.

SWEET POTATO FRIES:

One large sweet potato

1–2 teaspoons of olive oil

1 tablespoon of fresh rosemary, chopped

Pinch of Celtic salt

FRIES PREP: Preheat the oven to 450° F. Wash and peel the sweet potato. Cut it up into fries. Take a thin non-stick baking pan and sprinkle with oil. Spread the fries in the pan and sprinkle with rosemary and salt. Bake until the fries become soft and slightly crunchy on the outside, turning them occasionally. Cooking time should take about 15 minutes.

WEDNESDAY

BREAKFAST 7:00–9:00 AM

Dr. Aviv Smoothie pH 5.96 | **F** | Serves 1

1 handful of ice cubes
½ cup of almond milk
1 cup of blueberries or mixed berries
1 banana

Blend thoroughly and drink up.

Notes: The almond milk neutralizes the acidity of the berries.

Modifications and additions: Add handful of spinach to make Dr. Aviv's Berry Smoothie Blast! (pH 6.11).

Add 1 tablespoon of hemp protein to make **Dr. Aviv's Protein Smoothie** (pH 6.25).

MORNING Mini-Meal 10:00–11:00 AM

Hard Boiled Egg ⊞ | Serves 1

1 whole egg
Pinch of Celtic salt

Boil egg in water for 15 minutes, peel and salt to taste.

LUNCH 12:30–2:30 PM

Kale Wrap with Guac Tapenade

pH 6.4 | Ⓥ | Serves 1

2 to 3 leaves of fresh kale

⅓ of a cucumber, scooped out seeds, peeled, finely chopped

Handful of arugula

12 pitted Kalamata olives (drained of oil)

1 ripe whole Haas avocado

1 teaspoon fresh cilantro, finely chopped

Use food processor to mash up olives, avocado, and cilantro. Spread guac tapenade on kale leaves, add cucumber and arugula, roll up and enjoy.

AFTERNOON Mini-Meal 3:00–4:00 PM

Toast with Almond Butter Ⓝ | Serves 1

1 slice of whole grain bread

1 teaspoon of organic almond butter

Small drizzle of honey (optional)

Spread almond butter on toast and drizzle with honey.

DINNER 6:00–7:30 PM

Turkey Burgers with Arugula Ginger Salad

Ⓐ̲ₚ̲ | Serves 1

TURKEY BURGERS:

4 ½ oz. of ground turkey (about a palmful)

2 tablespoons of raw carrots, shredded

1 tablespoon of raw celery, shredded

3 tablespoons of zucchini, finely chopped (optional)

3 tablespoons of potatoes, shredded

1 small egg

¼ teaspoon of Celtic salt

2 tablespoons of whole wheat flour

1–2 sprays of Bragg Liquid Aminos (per burger)

1 teaspoon of olive oil

TURKEY BURGERS PREP: In a large bowl, mix all the shredded vegetables with the turkey and sprinkle with salt. In a different bowl, beat the egg and pour half of it over the turkey mix. (Be careful not to use all of the egg as the turkey might become too moist.) Mix the turkey and veggies completely and then make 3–4 burgers from the mixture. On another plate, pour out the flour and then coat each burger thoroughly.

Heat up the oil in a non-stick pan on low, then place the burgers in the pan and cover. Cook the burgers for approximately 4–5 minutes, turning them over occasionally. After burgers are cooked, turn off stove and spray each burger with 1–2 sprays of Bragg Liquid Aminos.

ARUGULA GINGER SALAD:

½ cup of finely chopped arugula

1 ½ cups of spinach

Carrot-ginger dressing (see recipe below)

CARROT-GINGER DRESSING: pH 5.73

4 tablespoons of raw carrots, shredded or chopped

1 tablespoon of olive oil

1 tablespoon of agave (sweetener)

¼ inch raw ginger, coarsely chopped

¼ teaspoon Celtic salt

¼ cup of water

CARROT-GINGER DRESSING PREP: Put all ingredients in food processor and mix until desired consistency is achieved.

SALAD PREP: Mix arugula and spinach, add dressing to taste.

BREAKFAST 7:00-9:00 AM

Broccoli Egg Omelet ⬜ | Serves 1

1 whole egg
2 egg whites
½ teaspoon of olive oil or coconut oil
1 handful of broccoli, chopped
1 teaspoon of parmesan cheese
1 slice of toasted whole grain bread

Wash and cut up broccoli. Heat up the oil in a frying pan on medium heat. Add broccoli and cook for about a minute. Add eggs and parmesan cheese and stir slightly until eggs are fluffy. When the eggs are cooked to your liking, turn off flame and serve with one slice of toasted whole grain bread.

MORNING Mini-Meal 10:00-11:00 AM

Fresh Fruit 8 oz. ⬜ | Serves 1

8 oz. of fresh fruit

Choose from cantaloupe, papaya, watermelon, honeydew, ripe Bosc pear, banana, or lychee.

Vegetable Pasta Salad ⓥ | Serves 1

½ cup of whole grain fusilli pasta

5–6 stalks of asparagus

3 oz. of Cremini mushrooms

1 handful of fresh arugula, roughly chopped

2 teaspoons of parmesan cheese

1 teaspoon of olive oil

1 tablespoon of fresh parsley, chopped

Celtic salt

In a sauce pan, heat up 2 cups of water and add a pinch of salt. Add pasta to the boiling water and cook for approximately 9 minutes. Wash the asparagus, break off about an inch from the end of each stalk, then cut into ½ inch segments. Clean, then slice mushrooms into chunks. Put the oil in a frying pan and turn the heat to medium. Add the mushrooms, asparagus, chopped parsley, and pinch of salt. Sauté for about 3 minutes, stirring occasionally. Remove the vegetables from the pan and mix into pasta. Add the chopped arugula and parmesan cheese, mix well, and enjoy a wonderful vegetarian pasta meal.

AFTERNOON Mini-Meal 3:00–4:00 PM

Assorted Tree Nuts Ⓝ | Serves 1

1 oz. (about a handful) of your choice

Mix from walnuts, cashews, pecans, and pistachios.

DINNER 6:00–7:30 PM

Fish & Chips 🔲 | Serves 1

5–6 oz. fillet of fish (tilapia, trout, flounder, branzino, sole)

1 large sweet potato

2 teaspoons of fresh rosemary, chopped

2 thin slices of lemon

2–3 teaspoons of olive oil

Pinch of Celtic salt

FISH PREP: Preheat oven to 400° F. Place a sheet of aluminum foil, about double the size of the fish fillet, on a non-stick baking pan. Sprinkle it with olive oil and place the fish on the foil. Season it with salt and one teaspoon of chopped rosemary. Place the lemon slices on the fish and close the foil around the fish, creating a tight pocket.

FRIES PREP: Cut the sweet potato into thin fries. Pour about 2 teaspoons of olive oil around the fish-foil pocket. Place the fries in the pan surrounding the "fish-pocket" and sprinkle the fries with salt and the remaining rosemary.

FINAL PREP: Place the pan in the oven and cook for about 15 minutes. You should turn the fries with a spatula occasionally. When the fries become soft on the inside and a bit crunchy on the outside, turn off the oven and pull out the pan. The fish should be tender and separate into pieces easily.

BREAKFAST 7:00–9:00 AM

Pear Oatmeal with Pecans & Coconut Flakes

G | Serves 1

5 tablespoons of old fashioned rolled oats

½ cup non-dairy milk (soy milk (non-GMO), almond milk, or rice milk)

½ soft ripe pear, cut into small chunks

1 teaspoon honey

Pinch of Celtic salt

1 tablespoon of fresh raw pecans (or walnuts), chopped

1 tablespoon coconut flakes

2–3 drops of vanilla extract

In a small saucepan, heat up the non-dairy milk and sea salt. Add oats and vanilla extract, and cook on medium, constantly stirring until thick and creamy, about 2–3 minutes. Remove from the stove and mix in the pear chunks, honey, pecans, and coconut flakes.

MORNING Mini-Meal 10:00–11:00 AM

Mozzarella Herb Toast V | Serves 1

1–2 thin slices of fresh mozzarella

2 leaves of fresh basil

1 slice of whole grain bread

Toast bread and place mozzarella and basil on bread.

Colorful Chicken Salad 🔲 | Serves 1

4–5 oz. chicken breast

3–4 oz. of corn (organic)

3–4 oz. green beans

1 teaspoon olive oil

SAUCE:

2–3 tablespoons of Bragg Liquid Aminos

1 tablespoon of honey

Sprinkle of Celtic salt (optional)

CHICKEN PREP: Preheat the oven to 450° F. Place the chicken in a pan and sprinkle with olive oil and a pinch of salt. Place the pan in the oven and roast for about 10–15 minutes, flipping the chicken occasionally. After cooked, let the chicken cool, then chop into small cubes.

VEGETABLE PREP (FRESH OR FROZEN): Cook corn kernels in boiling water until slightly tender, about 2 minutes. Drain the water from the corn, add green beans to fresh boiling water and cook for 1-2 minutes, maintaining the crunchiness of the beans. Drain the water from the beans, let slightly cool, then chop into half inch segments. If using frozen corn or green beans, defrost them by placing them in boiling water for about 1–2 minutes. Next, drain corn or green beans well, let them cool off for a few minutes, then chop the green beans finely.

SAUCE PREP: Blend the Bragg Liquid Aminos and honey together. Add a pinch of salt if necessary.

FINAL PREP: Combine the chicken and vegetables, then add the sauce, and mix it in well.

Modifications and additions: Once you have graduated successfully to the Sustainable Phase of the Acid Watcher® Diet, you can make an even more colorful version of this salad by adding:
½ roasted red pepper, chopped
2 tablespoons raw leeks, finely chopped

Fresh Fruit 5-6 oz. 🔲 | Serves 1

5–6 oz. of fresh fruit

Choose from cantaloupe, papaya, watermelon, honeydew, ripe Bosc pear, banana, or lychee.

Papaya Salad 🔲 | Serves 1

1 large kale leaf (about 12 inches), chopped
3 teaspoons of walnuts, finely chopped
3 heaping tablespoons of shredded carrots
⅓ of a cup of cucumbers, chopped
½ teaspoon of olive oil
10–15 raisins, chopped
2 tablespoons of crumbled feta cheese
½ cup of papaya (non-GMO), cut into ½ inch cubes
Carrot-ginger dressing (see recipe below)

CARROT-GINGER DRESSING: pH 5.7
4 tablespoons of raw carrots, shredded
1 tablespoon of olive oil
1 tablespoon of agave (sweetener)
¼ inch raw ginger, coarsely chopped
¼ teaspoon Celtic salt
¼ cup of water

CARROT-GINGER DRESSING PREP: Add all of the dressing ingredients into a food processor and blend well until the consistency is to your liking.

In a large bowl, blend all the salad ingredients, except for the papaya. Add 2–3 tablespoons of dressing and mix it in well. Top with papaya cubes.

BREAKFAST 7:00–9:00 AM

Green Juice (12–15 oz.) 🟥 | Serves 1

7 oz. large carrots (2-3)

4-5 oz. kale (5-6 leaves)

2 stalks of celery

1 ripe Bosc pear or ½ cup of any other fruit above pH 5

(please refer to Chapter 7)

1 cucumber

1 cup of spinach

Other optional ingredients are beets, bok choy, parsley, cilantro, Swiss chard, lettuce, spirulina powder.

Put all ingredients in a juicer and juice it. Once poured into a cup, add a few cubes of ice (if desired) and sip slowly. Feel free to combine these ingredients according to your own taste. In order to make the vegetable juice sweeter, add more carrots.

Notes: If you do not own a juicer, please go to a local store that makes fresh juice, choosing as close to the above ingredients as possible.

MORNING Mini-Meal 10:00–11:00 AM

Toast with Almond Butter and Honey 🟦 | Serves 1

1 slice of whole grain bread

½ teaspoon of almond butter

Drizzle of honey (optional)

Lightly toast bread and spread with almond butter, then drizzle with honey. Make sure you stick to one slice only.

Broiled Herb Salmon with Steamed Spinach

AP | Serves 1

5 oz. of salmon fillet

1 teaspoon herbs (fresh or dried parsley, thyme, sage, rosemary)

2 pinches of Celtic salt

Full cup of freshly washed spinach

1½ teaspoons of olive oil

½ cup of water

½ fresh lemon, sliced

SALMON PREP: Pour one teaspoon of olive oil in a pan on low to medium heat for about 1 minute, then pour ¼ of a cup of water into the pan and simmer. Place the salmon in the pan and add a pinch of salt, half the herbs, and several lemon slices to the salmon and cover. Continue to cook over medium heat.

Turn the salmon over after 2–3 minutes. Add the rest of the herbs and pinch of salt and cover. Be sure to add more water if the water evaporates before the salmon is cooked. Should you want the salmon crispier, cook it a little bit longer after all the water evaporates from the pan, keeping a watchful eye on it so it doesn't start to burn.

SPINACH PREP: Heat up ¼ cup of water in a frying pan. Add spinach and cover up. Sauté on low heat for 1 minute. Sprinkle with salt and stir. Remove from the pan and drain. Add ½ teaspoon of olive oil and serve.

OPTIONAL: Include ½ slice of toasted whole grain bread.

Fresh Fruit 8 oz. F | Serves 1

8 oz. of fresh fruit

Choose from cantaloupe, papaya, watermelon, honeydew, ripe pear, banana, or lychee.

DINNER 6:00–7:30 PM

Roasted Vegetable Sandwich 🔲 | Serves 2

½ medium yellow squash

½ sweet potato

2 slices of eggplant (½ inch thick)

2 slices of mozzarella cheese

4 fresh basil leaves

Pinch Celtic salt

1–2 teaspoons olive oil

2 slices of whole grain bread

1 egg (optional)

2 tablespoons of whole wheat flour (optional)

VEGETABLE PREP: Peel the yellow squash and cut it lengthwise into 4 slices. Wash and peel the sweet potato and slice it into 8 thin circular pieces that resemble chips. Cut two separate ½ inch thick slices of eggplant. (Vegetables left over can be saved in the refrigerator for one of your upcoming meals.)

Preheat oven to 450° F. Whisk the egg with a pinch of salt in a bowl. Dip the yellow squash into it to coat, then on a separate plate, pour out flour and completely cover squash with flour coating.

In a non-stick roasting pan, add 2 teaspoons of olive oil, spreading it out evenly. Place the yellow squash, sweet potato, and eggplant in the pan and season with salt.

Put in the oven and roast until the potatoes are soft, about 10–15 minutes. Flip the yellow squash and the rest of the vegetables a couple of times throughout the roasting process.

SANDWICH PREP: Lightly toast the bread and first add the cheese, then the basil, followed by the squash, potato, and finally the eggplant. Cover with another slice of bread and enjoy a truly delicious, healthy sandwich.

OPTIONS: Breading the yellow squash is optional. You can simply slice it and place in the roasting pan with the rest of the vegetables.

Modifications and additions: When you get to the Sustainable Phase of the Acid Watcher® Diet, you may add roasted red peppers.

Acid Watcher® Diet Healing Phase: **ADDITIONAL RECIPES**

For those of you who are more skillful in the kitchen or have more time to cook, below are some additional recipes that can be substituted for another meal within its particular Healing Phase meal plan food category, such as **AP** for another Animal Protein meal, or **F** for another Fruit meal. Please note that some of the following recipes will require additional ingredients not found in the Healing Phase Weekly Shopping List.

BREAKFAST

High Fiber Rice Pudding **G** | Serves 2

½ cup of brown rice
½ cup of soy milk
1½ tablespoons of honey
1½ tablespoons of shredded coconut
2 tablespoons of raisins
3–4 dried apricots, chopped
1 teaspoon of vanilla extract (optional)

Rinse the rice and boil it in a small pot until cooked, about 20 minutes. Drain rice of any water and add milk. Bring rice to a boil while stirring occasionally. Add the vanilla extract and cook for an additional few minutes. Turn off heat and stir in the honey, coconut, raisins, and apricots, then serve.

Mexican Shrimp Salad with Avocado, Black Beans, and Cilantro **AP** | Serves 2

½ lb. jumbo shrimp, cleaned and deveined

½ teaspoon Celtic salt (¼ teaspoon for shrimp + ¼ teaspoon for salad)

1 jumbo romaine heart, chopped

½ English cucumber, sliced

¾ cup of raw black beans (if from a can, the product must be organic)

1 avocado, sliced

3 teaspoons olive oil
   (1 teaspoon for the shrimp + 2 teaspoons for the vegetables)

2 tablespoons raw pepitas (pumpkin seeds)

½ cup cilantro, roughly chopped

BEAN PREP: Rinse 1 cup of dried black beans and clean thoroughly. Place the beans in a large bowl, cover with water, and let soak overnight. The next day, strain and rinse the beans, then put them in a medium saucepan and cover them with water. Add a big pinch of salt, bring to a boil, and reduce to a simmer with the lid on. Cook for about 40–50 minutes, or until soft, but not mushy. Drain and rinse well. Let cool.

It is all right to use beans from a can as long as the product is organic. The reason behind this is that non-organic canned products contain chemicals that should be avoided as much as possible, especially for acid reflux sufferers. Organic canned beans should only contain water, salt, and beans.

To use canned beans for this recipe, simply open the can, rinse the beans slightly, and add them to your meal.

VEGETABLE PREP: Mix and toss the romaine, cucumber, black beans, avocado, pepitas, cilantro, 2 teaspoons of olive oil, and ¼ teaspoon of salt.

SHRIMP/MEAL PREP: Heat a large sauté pan over a medium flame. In a bowl, toss the shrimp with ½ teaspoon of olive oil and ¼ teaspoon of salt. Add the shrimp to the pan in an even layer, add ½ teaspoon of oil, and sear until fully cooked, about 1–2 minutes per side. Place the vegetables on a plate, top with the shrimp and serve.

Acid Watcher® Nicoise Salad AP | Serves 2

2 x 4 oz. tuna steaks

1 jumbo Romaine heart, chopped

2 hardboiled eggs, peeled and cut up

4½ oz. green beans, trimmed,
   blanched, and chopped into ½ inch pieces

½ cup Kalamata olives, pitted

5 tablespoons of carrots, shredded

1 cup of cucumber, cut into half moons

⅓ cup basil, roughly chopped

¼ cup of parsley, chopped

2½ teaspoons olive oil
   (½ teaspoon for the fish + 2 teaspoons for the salad)

¼ teaspoon Celtic salt for the vegetables
   and a couple of dashes for the fish

TUNA PREP: Rub medium sauté pan with a cloth containing some olive oil, and heat over a medium flame. Sprinkle both sides of each tuna steak with Celtic salt and place in the hot pan. Sear for about 1 minute on each side, keeping the center rare. Remove from the heat and slice.

SALAD/MEAL PREP: Toss together the romaine, eggs, green beans, olives, carrots, cucumber, basil, parsley, teaspoon olive oil, and ¼ teaspoon of salt. Top with the seared tuna and serve.

Modifications and additions: For a vegetarian option, don't add tuna.

Salmon Spinach Salad with Sliced Pears, Walnuts, and Olives [AP] | Serves 2

2 x 4 oz. salmon fillets

4 cups baby spinach

1 soft/ripe medium Bosc pear, thinly sliced into ½ inch pieces

½ cup cooked chickpeas*

½ cup walnuts, toasted and roughly chopped

½ cup golden raisins

¼ cup Kalamata olives, pitted and chopped

¼ cup green olives, pitted

1 teaspoon olive oil, plus a little more for drizzling

¼ teaspoon Celtic salt

SALMON PREP: Place the salmon on a greased aluminum lined baking sheet, drizzle with olive oil, sprinkle with salt, and broil until golden brown, about 5–7 minutes.

CHICKPEA PREP: Rinse one cup of dried chickpeas, picking out any stones. Place the chickpeas in a large bowl and cover completely with water. Let soak overnight. The next day, strain and rinse them, then place in a medium sauce pan and cover with water. Add a big pinch of salt, bring to a boil, and reduce to a simmer with the lid on. Cook for about 40–50 minutes, or until soft, but not mushy. Drain and rinse well. Let cool.

*If you want to use chickpeas from a can, please make sure they are organic. Organic canned beans should only contain water, salt, and beans. To use canned beans for this recipe, simply open the can, rinse the beans, and add them to your meal.

FINAL PREP: Toss the spinach, pears, chickpeas, walnuts, raisins, olives, 1 tablespoon of olive oil, along with ¼ teaspoon of salt. Top with the salmon and serve.

Herb Chicken AP | Serves 2

2 teaspoons of olive oil

4 oz. of chicken breast

2 tablespoons of herbs (fresh or dried rosemary, oregano, parsley, thyme, sage)

Celtic salt for seasoning

½ teaspoon of paprika

Whole grain bread crumbs for sprinkling

Preheat the oven to 400° F. Slice the chicken into thin fillets. On a baking sheet, add the oil and spread out the chicken fillets. Sprinkle the fillets with salt, paprika, and herbs on both sides. Then coat chicken on both sides with the bread crumbs.

Roast for about 15 minutes. Chicken should be flipped over half-way through the roasting process. Serve with vegetables of your choice above pH 5, still keeping in mind that you should consume one pound of veggies every day.

Chicken Soup AP | Serves 4

1½ medium zucchini, chopped (5-6 oz.)

1 stalk of celery, chopped

½ cup of chopped carrots

1½ cups of potatoes, cut in cubes

6 oz. of chicken, cut in small cubes

2-3 tablespoons of green peas

1 teaspoon Celtic salt

1 teaspoon of olive oil

3 cups of organic vegetable broth

4 cups of water

Fresh parsley, to season

Paprika, to season

Heat up the oil in a pot and add chopped zucchini and celery. Stir for about a minute. Add 3 cups of broth and 3 cups of boiling hot water and cover up. Let it cook for about 10 minutes, then add carrots, potatoes, chicken, and 1 teaspoon of Celtic salt. Cook until the chicken and potatoes are almost done, approximately 10 minutes. Add the green peas, chopped parsley, sprinkle with paprika and a bit more water if necessary. Cook for an additional couple of minutes then remove from the stove, let it cool a bit, then serve.

Roasted Beets and Fresh Cucumber with Creamy White Bean Dip V | Serves 2

1 bunch of small red beets (approximately 4 small beets),
   roasted and cut into rounds
1 cucumber, sliced
1 cup cannellini beans*
¼ cup water
2½ teaspoons of olive oil
   (2 teaspoons for the beets + ½ teaspoon for the bean dip)
¾ teaspoon of Celtic salt
   (¼ teaspoon for the beets + ½ teaspoon for the bean dip)
1 tablespoon of fresh dill, finely chopped

BEETS PREP: Preheat oven to 350° F. Wash, trim, and dry the beets. Cut them in half for quicker cooking and place them on a large sheet of aluminum foil. Add 2 teaspoons olive oil and ¼ teaspoon of salt. Rub in the oil and salt and evenly coat. Wrap the aluminum tightly around the beets. Place on a baking sheet and roast until fork tender, about 20–30 minutes, depending on the size of the beets. Let them cool, then rub a paper towel over them to remove the skins, then slice into rounds.

CANNELLINI BEAN PREP: Rinse 1 cup of dried cannellini beans and clean thoroughly. Place the beans in a large bowl and cover with water. Let soak overnight. The next day, strain and rinse them, then place in a medium sauce pan and cover with water. Add a big pinch of salt, bring to a boil, and reduce to a simmer with the lid on. Cook for about 40–50 minutes, or until soft, but not mushy. Drain and rinse well. Let cool.

*Again, if you want to use beans from a can, please make sure the product is organic. Organic canned beans should only contain water, salt, and beans. To use canned beans for this recipe, just open the can, rinse the beans slightly, and add to recipe.

FINAL PREP: Place the cannellini beans in a food processor with the water, olive oil, and salt. Purée until smooth, then stir in the dill. Serve with the sliced beets and cucumbers.

Beet and Quinoa Salad with Steamed Kale and Chickpeas Ⓥ | Serves 2

1 bunch of beets (approximately 4 small beets)

1 cup quinoa, cooked

½ bunch Lacinato kale (approximately 10 leaves),
  deribbed and thinly sliced

½ cup chickpeas

¼ cup pine nuts

3½ teaspoons of olive oil
  (2 teaspoons for the beets + 1½ teaspoons for the salad)

½ teaspoon of Celtic salt (¼ teaspoon for the beets
  and ¼ teaspoon for the quinoa + seasoning)

2 thin slices of lemon

ROASTED BEET PREP (SAME AS BEFORE): Preheat oven to 350° F. Wash, trim, and dry the beets. Cut them in half, then place them on a large sheet of aluminum foil. Add 2 teaspoons of olive oil and ¼ teaspoon of salt. Rub in the oil and salt and coat evenly. Wrap the aluminum tightly around the beets. Place on a baking sheet and roast until fork tender, about 20–30 minutes depending on the size of the beets. Let them cool, then rub a paper towel over them to remove the skins, then chop into ¼ inch pieces.

QUINOA PREP: Boil 1¼ cups of water with ¼ teaspoon Celtic salt. Pour in 1 cup quinoa, reduce heat to low, and cover. Simmer until water is absorbed and quinoa is tender and fluffy, about 15 minutes. Turn off flame but keep the lid on and let sit for 5 minutes.

CHICKPEA PREP: Rinse 1 cup of dried chickpeas, picking out any stones. Place the chickpeas in a large bowl and cover completely with water. Let soak overnight. The next day, strain and rinse the chickpeas, then place them in a medium sauce pan, and cover with water. Add a big pinch of salt, bring to a boil, and reduce to a simmer with the lid on. Cook for about 40–50 minutes, or until soft, but not mushy. Drain and rinse well. Let cool.

If you want to use chickpeas from a can, please make sure the product is organic. Organic canned beans should only contain water, salt, and beans. To use canned chickpeas for this recipe, just open the can, rinse the beans slightly, and add to recipe.

KALE PREP: In a medium saucepan, heat up ¼ cup of water. Keep the heat low and add the chopped kale, dash of salt, and lemon slices. Cover up and let soften for a couple minutes, making sure that the kale still retains some crunch. Drain the excess water, remove the lemon slices, and let cool.

FINAL PREP: Combine the beets, cooked quinoa, kale, chickpeas, pine nuts, 1½ teaspoons of olive oil, and another touch of salt (if desired).

Puréed Butternut Squash Soup with Seared Mushrooms & Herbs 🔳 | Serves 2

1 butternut squash, peeled and cut into 1 inch cubes

1 teaspoon dried thyme

1½ teaspoons of Celtic salt (for squash) + sprinkle (for mushrooms)

2½ cups water

½ cup non-dairy milk (soy milk (non-GMO), almond milk, or rice milk)

8 oz. of Cremini mushrooms,
   stemmed and halved or sliced, depending on the size

2-3 tablespoons parsley, chopped

2-3 teaspoons olive oil

SOUP PREP: Heat the olive oil in a large pot over a medium flame. Add the butternut squash, dried thyme, 1½ teaspoons of Celtic salt, and sauté until browned and fragrant, about 10 minutes. Pour in the water, bring it to a boil, then cover up and simmer the squash until it becomes tender, about 10 more minutes. Add the non-dairy milk.

Transfer the squash along with all of its liquid to a blender and purée until smooth, about 2 minutes.

MUSHROOM PREP: Heat 2-3 teaspoons of olive oil in a large sauté pan over a high flame. Once the oil is simmering, add the mushrooms in an even layer but do not stir. Let them get golden brown, about 4 minutes, then mix. Cook 3-5 minutes longer and sprinkle with salt. Transfer to a paper towel-lined plate.

FINAL PREP: To serve, top the butternut squash soup with the seared mushrooms and sprinkle with chopped parsley.

Asian Steamed Spinach with Raw Sesame Seeds

V | Serves 2

2 tablespoons Bragg Liquid Aminos (BLA)

11 oz. fresh baby spinach

Handful raw sesame seeds

In a medium saucepan, heat the BLA over a medium-high flame until it starts to steam. Add the baby spinach and let the steaming BLA wilt the spinach. Toss to distribute the heat evenly. Top with sesame seeds and serve.

Watermelon Mozzarella Cocktail

pH 5.35 | **F** | Serves 1

10 x 1 inch cubes of watermelon

1 slice of fresh Buffalo mozzarella, cut up

2 leaves of basil, chopped

Pinch of Celtic salt

Place watermelon, mozzarella, and basil in a bowl. Toss gently, then sprinkle with salt.

Cantaloupe Express pH 5.72 | **F** | Serves 1

6 tablespoons of cantaloupe

1 slice of Buffalo mozzarella, cut up

2 small sprigs of savory, chopped

2 small sprigs of rosemary, chopped

Pinch of Celtic salt

Place watermelon, mozzarella, and chopped herbs in a bowl. Toss gently, then sprinkle with salt.

PHASE 2 OF THE ACID WATCHER® DIET: THE SUSTAINABLE PHASE

After the four-week Healing Phase of the Diet is completed, the **Sustainable Phase** of the Acid Watcher® Diet begins. Please note that the Sustainable Phase also has its list of "non-negotiables" which must be adhered to or you run the risk of having your acid reflux return.

The Acid Watcher® Diet Sustainable Phase "Non-Negotiables"

1. **NO** food or beverages less than pH 4
2. **NO** alcohol
3. **NO** lying down within three hours after eating
4. **NO** carbonated beverages (including all sugary sodas, club soda, or sparkling water)
5. **NO** caffeine
6. **NO** prepackaged (processed) foods
7. **NO** deep-fried food
8. **NO** chocolate
9. **NO** food with mint (including gum)
10. **NO** smoking of any substance

The Sustainable Phase of the Acid Watcher® Diet (see Figure 8.2) is the type of diet you will essentially be on for the rest of your life, if you want to avoid your acid reflux from making an unwanted return. This second phase of the Diet adheres to the same type of meal plan as the Healing Phase, namely, the **eating schedule**, **portion sizes**, and **food preparation rules** stay *exactly the same*. The only adjustment is that the Sustainable Phase allows for foods that have a pH level down to 4, whereas the four-week Healing Phase allowed only for foods above pH 5.

Take-out Corner

The Sustainable Phase of the Acid Watcher® Diet also has its list of "non-negotiables" which must be adhered to or you run the risk of having your acid reflux return.

Although the list of additional foods is not very long, it will be a nice addition to your already established Acid Watcher® Diet program. When you introduce new food items, do it gradually so that you are able to observe how that particular food affects you.

Please note that some of these "new foods" have already appeared in the Healing Phase of the Diet. What made those particular foods permissible during your initial Healing Phase was that I combined them with much higher pH foods to create a meal that was more alkaline and therefore safe for you.

It is very important to note that if you find that any of the foods listed below becomes a "trigger food" for you, causing even the slightest reflux symptom, you must avoid it. Lastly, please keep in mind that pH levels can vary depending on the ripeness, freshness, or source of the product. Ripe fruits and vegetables tend to have a higher pH level than those that are not fully ripe.

The Acid Watcher® Diet Sustainable Phase:
FOODS THAT CAN NOW BE ADDED TO YOUR DIET

Fruit

Kiwi	pH 4.84
Mango	pH 4.58
Figs	pH 4.55
Apples (Golden Delicious)	pH 4.50
Cherries	pH 4.43
Raisins (dark)	pH 4.41
Prunes (dried)	pH 4.27
Peaches (yellow, ripe)	pH 4.25
Blueberries (now can be consumed without the aid of other neutralizing foods such as almond milk)	pH 4.19
Grapes (green, seedless)	pH 4.12

Note: The ideal way to introduce the new fruit items is through your daily morning or afternoon Mini-Meals.

(continued on next page)

(continued from previous page)

Vegetables
Leeks   pH 6.21

Bell Peppers   pH 4.8–5.2

Note: You may add leeks and peppers to the *Colorful Chicken Salad*, or any salad or side dish. However, please keep in mind that leeks and peppers are carminatives, which means that there is the possibility that they might loosen your LES (lower esophageal sphincter). This is why I had you avoid them during the initial Healing Phase of the Diet.

Dairy
Feta cheese   pH 4.6

Yogurt (plain, Stonefield)   pH 4.43

Kefir   pH 4.17

Note: Yogurt can become one of your main new breakfast options.

Figure 8.2
Acid Watcher® Diet: Weekly Sustainable Phase
Sample Meal Plan

	SUNDAY	MONDAY	TUESDAY	WEDNESDAY	THURSDAY	FRIDAY	SATURDAY
BREAKFAST 7–9 AM	(F) Pineapple Express Smoothie	(ED) Yogurt with Raisins and Almonds	(G) Acid Watcher® Blueberry Crêpes	(F) Dr. Aviv Smoothie	(ED) Spinach Omelet	(G) Pear Oatmeal	(V) Green Juice
MORNING MINI-MEAL 10–11 AM	(V) Guac Tapenade Toast	(F) Fresh Fruit 8 oz.	(V) Raw Veggies	(ED) Hard Boiled Egg	(F) Fresh Fruit 8 oz.	(ED) Mozzarella Herb Toast	(N) Toast with Almond Butter & Honey
LUNCH 12–2:30 PM	(AP) Mexican Shrimp Salad	(V) High Fiber Salad	(AP) Pesto Chicken Sandwich	(V) Kale Wrap	(V) Vegetable Pasta Salad	(AP) Colorful Chicken Salad	(AP) Stuffed Baked Salmon with Sweet Potato
AFTERNOON MINI-MEAL 3–4 PM	(NF) Dr. Aviv Power Bar	(N) Assorted Tree Nuts	(F) Fresh Fruit 6–7 oz.	(NF) Almond Butter & Banana	(N) Assorted Tree Nuts	(F) Fresh Fruit 5–6 oz.	(F) Peach Blossom Smoothie
DINNER 6–7:30 PM	(V) Kale Salad	(AP) Miso Halibut with Bok Choy	(V) Brussels Sprout Salad with Pecans, Raisins, and Apple	(AP) Turkey Burger with Arugula Salad	(AP) Broiled Fish and Vegetables	(V) Papaya Salad	(V) Puréed Butternut Squash Soup with Seared Mushrooms

(AP) =Animal Protein, (ED) =Eggs or Dairy, (F) =Fruit, (G) =Grain, (NF) =Nut-based, (N) =Nuts and Fruit, (V) =Vegetarian

The Acid Watcher® Diet Sustainable Phase: **RECIPES**

Acid Watcher® Blueberry Crêpes   G | Serves 2

1 cup of whole grain flour

1¼ cups of almond milk

½ cup of water

Drizzle of either olive oil or coconut oil

1 egg

Pinch of Celtic salt

Pinch of raw (unprocessed) sugar

Sprinkle of vanilla extract (optional)

FILLING:

1 cup of blueberries

2 teaspoons of raw (unprocessed) sugar

CRÊPE PREP: In a large bowl, mix the flour, 1 cup of almond milk, 1 cup of water, egg, salt, sugar, and vanilla. Mix well with a whisk or electric blender. To achieve the right thickness, you may add several more tablespoons of milk or water.

In a medium frying pan, add a few drops of olive oil or coconut oil on medium heat. Use a ladle to spread out batter in pan. The best way to spread out the batter is to lift up the pan from the stove and slowly pour the batter, starting at the top of the pan while tilting it around to allow the batter to spread evenly in a thin layer. Once spread out evenly, place the pan back on the stove and cook the crêpe for a couple of minutes. Loosen the edges of the crêpe by using a thin flat spatula, flip the crêpe, and cook for several minutes more.

After the crêpe is cooked and moved onto a plate, simply repeat the process until all of the crêpe batter is used up. Ideally you should use a non-stick pan at least until you become proficient in crêpe making. It is not necessary to add oil in between every crêpe you make because as a reflux sufferer, the less oil you use when cooking, the better.

FILLING PREP: In a medium saucepan, add about 8 oz. of fresh blueberries and 2 teaspoons of raw (unprocessed) sugar. Mix well and bring to a boil. Slightly mash the blueberries with a spatula to help them release their juice. After a couple of minutes, remove from the stove.

FINAL PREP: Take one crêpe and add a tablespoon of the filling to the middle. Wrap it up either into triangles or the way you would wrap a burrito or blintz. Repeat the process with the remaining crêpes and filling.

Yogurt with Raisins and Almonds ⊞ | Serves 2

3 tablespoons of plain, regular yogurt

½ banana

2 teaspoons of raisins

1 teaspoon of raw almonds or walnuts, ground

Honey (small splash if necessary)

Add fruit and nuts to yogurt. Stir and serve.

Smoothies F

(All smoothies are prepared in a blender)

Papaya Chill pH 4.77 | Serves 1

1 cup of papaya cut into small cubes

2 tablespoons of plain regular yogurt

½ of a banana

½ cup of ice

*Pineapple Express pH 4.47 | Serves 1

½ cup of pineapple

½ cup of papaya

½ banana

⅓ cup of soy milk

Handful of ice

*Pineapple is acidic but when mixed with other ingredients in proper proportion, as in this smoothie, the acidity is neutralized.

Peach Blossom pH 4.52 | Serves 1

1 peach

1 mango

1 small banana

1 tablespoon of plain yogurt

½ teaspoon of vanilla extract

Handful of ice

Tropic Thunder pH 4.84 | Serves 1

1 small mango

½ cup of papaya

3–4 lychees

½ dragon fruit

½ banana

1 tablespoon of yogurt

½ cup of ice

Brussels Sprout Salad with Pecans, Raisins, and Apple Ⓥ | Serves 2

1 lb. Brussels sprouts, trimmed, and sliced

1 apple, cored, and thinly sliced/chopped into ½ inch pieces

½ cup raw pecans, chopped

½ cup raisins

2 teaspoons olive oil (1 teaspoon for Brussels sprout prep. + 1 teaspoon for seasoning of salad)

Celtic salt to season

BRUSSELS SPROUTS PREP: Preheat oven to 350° F. Trim and slice the Brussels sprouts. Spread them out in a baking sheet and sprinkle with salt. Place them in the oven and roast for about 10–15 minutes. They should still stay crunchy and slightly toasted on the outside.

FINAL PREP: Toss Brussels sprouts along with all fruit and nuts together, season with olive oil and salt, and serve.

Stuffed Baked Salmon with Sweet Potato

AP | Serves 1

5–6 oz. salmon fillet

2–3 tablespoons of leeks, finely chopped

2 slices of lemon

2 teaspoons of olive oil

2 teaspoons of fresh rosemary, chopped

½ sweet potato

2–3 teaspoons of Bragg Liquid Aminos

Sprinkle of Celtic salt

SALMON PREP: Slice the salmon fillet in the middle, lengthwise, as if to make a sandwich. Sprinkle with salt on top and inside where you made the cut. Stuff it with leeks and pour two teaspoons of Bragg Liquid Aminos over the leek stuffing. Place the lemon slices on top of the leeks and close the salmon. Sprinkle the top with rosemary.

Preheat oven to 450° F. Drizzle an aluminum foil sheet with a teaspoon of olive oil and place it on a baking pan. Lay fish on the oiled foil and place in the oven.

SWEET POTATO PREP: Slice up the sweet potato into thin circles resembling chips. Sprinkle another teaspoon of oil in the pan around the aluminum foil. Spread the potatoes in the pan and place the pan in the oven. Bake until the fish and the potatoes are cooked, approximately 15 minutes. You should turn the potatoes over about halfway through the cooking process. No need to flip the fish over.

When cooked, pull it out of the oven and sprinkle the fish with one more teaspoon of Bragg Liquid Aminos, then serve.

9

CLOSING THOUGHTS

*"When it comes to the health of my patients,
I always worry about what I can't see."*
—JONATHAN AVIV, MD, FACS

My medical career, which started nearly 30 years ago, has primarily been spent focusing on an issue that, although incredibly important in our lives, is often taken for granted. It's an area of our bodies that sits at the crossroads of sound, taste, and life itself. The intersection of where we eat and where we breathe. I'm referring to swallowing.

Since my days in medical school, I've always been fascinated by the swallowing region in our bodies—its complexity, its sensitivity, and of course, its unforgiving importance.

Earlier in my career as a head and neck surgeon, I routinely performed 15-hour, micro-vascular facial reconstructive surgeries. The surgeries usually followed the same basic outline. First, I would excise the cancerous tissue from the affected region in the head and neck. Then, I would reconstruct the patient's jaw, tongue, or throat when necessary by dissecting, and then transferring, flaps of skin and muscle from all over the body to the face and neck region.

Although the main objective during these long surgeries was to successfully remove the cancer, the patient usually faced a post-operative issue that even today is still not adequately addressed. What I'm alluding to is that often times these surgeries adversely affected a patient's ability to swallow normally.

In order to have a normal swallow, not only does motor function (how things *move*) in the head and neck have to be intact, but sensory function (how things *feel*) must be intact as well. Yet, after cancer surgery in the head and neck, both motor and sensory functions are often necessarily altered. This can lead to a patient choking and developing aspiration pneumonia.

Remarkably, as late as the early 1990s, all tests of swallowing function (pre-op or post-op) *only examined motor function*. There was no test available to assess *sensory function* in the head and neck, which is one of the most important predictors of a safe swallow. In other words, to solely examine motor function misses the complete physiologic picture of the patient.

As a result of the need to assess sensation during swallowing, I developed FEESST (Flexible Endoscopic Evaluation of Swallowing with Sensory Testing), a method and device which measures sensitivity in the throat. The assessment of swallowing function not only had application to determine my patient's post-operative swallowing status, but also had relevance in many other areas of medicine where swallowing impairment took place. This includes acute stroke, as well as diseases such as Parkinson, Multiple Sclerosis, Amyotrophic Lateral Sclerosis (Lou Gehrig's disease), as well as other chronic neurological conditions.

While performing FEESST on patients, whether with chronic neurological diseases or post-operative patients recovering from head and neck cancer operations, I noticed that their condition was often exacerbated by the swelling of their larynx due to acid reflux damage. By treating the acid reflux problem, I found that their swallowing problems began to improve.

Over the course of the next few years, following my development of FEESST (1993), I began to notice a dramatic increase in the overall number of patients who were experiencing acid reflux but went undiagnosed until I performed the FEESST procedure on them. As a result, FEESST became important in diagnosing severe cases of Throatburn Reflux where swallowing and throat sensitivity had been drastically impaired. Thus, a procedure that was originally intended to measure sensation in a person's throat became a diagnostic tool to detect acid reflux disease.

As I started to publish papers on FEESST, as well as on the connection between acid reflux and swallowing problems, I began to notice a marked increase in the incidence of esophageal cancer that was caused not by smoking and excessive drinking, but by acid reflux disease.

Although the linkage between acid reflux disease and esophageal cancer had previously been established, the extreme rate of growth was alarming. Esophageal cancer has been surpassing every other cancer in the U.S. and Europe since the mid-1970s.

It is imperative that we understand as soon as possible the importance of educating people about two things with respect to esophageal cancer—*new alarm symptoms* and *new diagnostic techniques*. The new alarm symptoms that can herald esophageal cancer are throat symptoms such as cough, hoarseness, throat clearing, and a lump-like sensation in the throat. The diagnostic technique that is available is not only sedated endoscopy (that we are all used to), but also **un**sedated endoscopy, a technique I pioneered called TransNasal Esophagoscopy (TNE).

A NEW TIDE IS HERE

It is my hope and belief that creating such awareness will lead to a **Targeted Individual Diagnostic Effort** (TIDE). This will direct patients with these new alarm symptoms to see their doctor, where a safe and inexpensive way to have their esophagus examined, such as TNE, can then take place. As patients with new alarm symptoms (throat symptoms) get examined, my hope is that we can stop esophageal cancer's rising trend and ultimately begin to reverse its course.

Spreading this extremely important message has become my personal crusade, and one that I intend to continue until the perception that acid reflux is innocuous, changes.

My desire to understand the physiology of a normal swallow and to heal people so they could eat and live normally, even when plagued by a terrible disease such as head and neck cancer, has been the foundation of my lifelong professional commitment.

I trust that you will follow the Acid Watcher® Diet detailed in this book. Please understand and follow the basic and important guidelines as they have been laid out for you. Namely, be sure to eat a diet that consists of low-acid foods balanced with natural macronutrients along with a high fiber component.

Good luck on your journey following a healthy diet, which will lead you to the healthy body you deserve. These aren't just words. This is a prescription that may one day save your life.

APPENDIX A:
True Patient Stories About Throatburn Reflux

"The poets did well to conjoin music and medicine, because the office of medicine is but to tune the curious harp of man's body."
—FRANCIS BACON, SR.

Hoarseness: Case #1

INITIAL PATIENT PRESENTATION

Jennifer, a 41-year-old clothing store manager, was complaining of worsening hoarseness over the last year.

PATIENT HISTORY/COMPLAINTS

The reason Jennifer came in to see me was that her hoarseness was getting in the way of her work. It got so bad that it was hard for customers to understand her because her voice was so raspy. Although Jennifer was in good outward physical shape, when she spoke, her voice was breathy, as if air was escaping beyond her control. She told me that her friends said she sounded like the Don Corleone character from the movie *The Godfather*. I asked Jennifer about her diet and lifestyle. She was a lifetime non-smoker. She occasionally ate dinner around 10 PM and went to sleep right afterwards. She didn't drink coffee or tea, rarely ate chocolate, seldom had alcohol, and only on occasion ate spicy foods. She never had heartburn, abdominal pain, or nausea. She also never had an upper gastrointestinal endoscopy. However, she mentioned that for the past several years, she drank two to three 16 oz. bottles of Coca-Cola, every day during her work week.

INITIAL EXAMINATION FINDINGS

Jennifer had a normal head and neck physical examination. I then examined her larynx with a specialized camera that allowed me to send a strobe light through the lens so that I could assess vocal fold vibration. It's a version of TFL (Transnasal Flexible Laryngoscopy, see Chapter 4) called Laryngeal Video Stroboscopy, or simply, Strobe. The Strobe exam of her larynx revealed severe damage in her throat and vocal folds. Her vocal folds, instead of being white, thin, and vibrating easily, looked like overcooked sausages—stiff and barely vibrating. She also had polyps on both sides of her vocal folds. The area of her larynx, close to where the esophagus begins, was as swollen as a golf ball (see Chapter 2 Figure 2.1 Normal and Acid Injured Larynx).

EXPLANATION OF FINDINGS TO THE PATIENT

I explained to Jennifer that she had severe acid reflux disease, the Throat-burn Reflux type. I further mentioned that the likely cause of her hoarseness was acid injury from two sources—her late night eating immediately followed by her lying down, and her frequent, prodigious consumption of highly acidic Coke (pH 2.5). When she asked me if she could possibly substitute Diet Coke for regular Coke, I explained that Diet Coke is also extremely acidic with a pH of 3.21, so definitely not.

TREATMENT PLAN

I treated Jennifer with a combination of the Acid Watcher® Diet and, initially, twice a day proton pump inhibitor (PPI) medication. I also encouraged Jennifer to see a speech language pathologist to help teach her how to take some of the strain away from her vocal folds. I asked

Jennifer to see me again in six weeks where I would also examine her esophagus with a TNE (TransNasal Esophagoscopy). In addition to re-examining her larynx, I explained that I was concerned that her chronic soda drinking could injure her esophagus as well as her larynx, and further discussed that it could take several months for her larynx swelling to return to normal.

FOLLOW UP #1

Six weeks later, Jennifer returned to my office with her voice slightly less hoarse, though still quite raspy. She had yet to see the speech therapist, but had cut down her late night eating and eliminated the Coca-Cola from her diet. She reported losing six pounds on the Acid Watcher® Diet as well. I performed a TNE and saw that her vocal folds were vibrating much better, and the redness and swelling of her vocal folds were much improved. The vocal fold polyps had shrunk by half, but were still there. Upon entering her esophagus, there was slight redness, but no evidence of Barrett esophagus. I did identify a small hiatal hernia (a portion of her stomach was above the diaphragm). Biopsies of the gastroesophageal junction, the area where the esophagus ends and the stomach begins, were performed. I advised Jennifer to continue both her antacid regimen and the Acid Watcher® Diet and have her larynx be examined again in six weeks. I emphasized the need to see the speech language pathologist to help treat her vocal fold polyps.

FOLLOW UP #2

Six weeks later, Jennifer returned for another examination of her larynx. Biopsies of her esophagus were negative for Barrett. This time her voice was vastly improved. She had seen the speech language pathologist for voice therapy and was staying off soda. The occasional late night meal had crept back into her lifestyle. On laryngeal exam, her vocal folds were now much less swollen, almost normal, with disappearance of her vocal fold polyps on both vocal folds. She had her voice back, she could be heard again, and she was quite happy with the results. She was astounded that the soft drink she had been consuming could have had such a profound negative affect on her voice and vocal folds. She was also surprised that in the absence of heartburn, she could still have acid reflux disease.

TAKE HOME MESSAGE

Consumption of carbonated, sugary sodas are devastating to the larynx. Their highly acidic nature activates pepsin receptors in the throat. When the sodas also contain caffeine, they also loosen the Lower Esophageal Sphincter (LES). However, Jennifer's injury was reversible with proper diet, lifestyle change, physical therapy (voice therapy given by the speech language pathologist), and antacid medication.

Hoarseness: Case #2

INITIAL PATIENT PRESENTATION

Joanie, a 38-year-old second grade teacher, was complaining of hoarseness for the past two years.

PATIENT HISTORY/COMPLAINTS

Joanie had been a professional a cappella singer for years before deciding to go back to teaching. She was one of two teachers in a class of 27 second graders. Joanie had been teaching for about two years while continuing to pursue singing as a hobby. About one year ago, she noticed that her voice would begin to fade, or get weaker, by the end of her work day. However, during the three weeks prior to seeing me, her voice started to fatigue by *lunchtime*. She drank two large cups of iced coffee every morning and never had time for breakfast. There was a delicious pizzeria around the corner from her school, so a slice of cheese pizza and a garden salad with oil and vinegar dressing was a lunchtime staple. She had singing practice three nights per week, so she didn't get home until after 10 PM each of those nights. Understandably, her late night music commitment meant that she didn't eat dinner until after 10 PM on those nights. She never had heartburn, she drank alcohol socially, primarily on weekends, and was an occasional chocolate eater and breath mint user. She rarely ate fried foods and was a lifetime non-smoker. She had no history of stomach ulcer, abdominal pain, or nausea.

INITIAL EXAMINATION FINDINGS

I performed a head and neck physical examination on Joanie and it was normal. A Strobe exam of the larynx was performed which showed the entire larynx to be swollen. The vocal folds themselves were not only swollen with diminished vibration, but there was a bump on each side of her vocal fold. The right vocal fold bump was twice the size of her left vocal fold bump.

EXPLANATION OF FINDINGS TO THE PATIENT

Normally, when one talks or sings, the vocal folds come together completely. But when there is a bump or a mass on the vocal fold, the vocal folds can't close entirely. Think of it as a large pebble separating the right and left sides of the vocal folds. In Joanie's case, the reason one bump was larger than the other was that one of the vocal folds had a tiny cyst within the vocal fold muscle. That little cyst kept slamming against the other vocal fold until the normal vocal fold started to show swelling as well. When there are two bumps in the vocal folds, typically one of the bumps is the actual disease process (a cyst, a blood clot, a piece of scar tissue) and the other side is a "reactive" process, meaning it had reacted to the constant trauma of having the bumped or spiked vocal fold hitting it. Imagine the normal vocal fold being "towel snapped" by the abnormal vocal fold.

TREATMENT PLAN

Joanie's treatment consisted of getting on the Acid Watcher® Diet. This included cutting out coffee, as well as pizza and vinegar. In addition, the late night eating routine had to be altered. Furthermore, speech therapy with a speech language pathologist was urged. I also prescribed two types of antacid medications—a PPI twice a day and a nighttime antacid called ranitidine (brand name Zantac) that complements the twice daily PPI. Because of Joanie's two years of hoarseness, I was concerned about her esophagus, so I asked her to return to my office in eight weeks to not only re-examine her larynx, but for a TNE as well.

FOLLOW UP #1

Eight weeks later, Joanie's voice was much improved and the daytime voice fatigue she had experienced had gone away. While performing TNE, I examined her larynx and saw that her primary lesion on the right vocal fold was still there, but much smaller. The lesion previously seen on the left vocal fold, the presumed "reactive" process, was now gone. From the laryngeal area, I continued into the esophagus. It showed some mild inflammation at the bottom of the esophagus without any evidence of Barrett. I then looked at the top of the stomach and it was normal. In addition, I performed biopsies of the inflamed areas of the esophagus. Because of the improved laryngeal exam and the minimal esophageal inflammation, I asked Joanie to stop the evening PPI and to continue the bedtime ranitidine. I advised her to continue with her speech therapy. Joanie figured out a way to eat before her singing practice so she would stop eating late at night before going to sleep. I reminded her to continue on with the Sustainable Phase of the Acid Watcher® Diet and asked her to return in six weeks.

FOLLOW UP #2

Six weeks later, on the second follow-up exam, Joanie's voice was back to normal. Biopsies of her esophagus were negative for Barrett. When Strobing the larynx, the primary vocal fold lesion had disappeared.

TAKE HOME MESSAGE

Caffeine, onion, and garlic have a physiological effect on the LES by loosening it. This causes the stomach contents to back up into the esophagus or the throat. This situation is made worse if a person eats late at night and goes to sleep right after dinner as the positive effect of being upright, using gravity to keep food in the stomach, is taken away once someone lies down. In addition, tomato sauce, due to its acidity, can also injure the esophagus on the way *down* into the stomach after a swallow, mainly because it can activate those pepsin receptors already present in the esophagus.

Hoarseness: Case #3

INITIAL PATIENT PRESENTATION

Albert, a 58-year-old voice-over actor, was unable to reach his upper register for the last three months.

PATIENT HISTORY/COMPLAINTS

Albert performs different types of voice-over jobs, from commercials to audio books. He was currently auditioning for a series of commercials, but for the past three months had been having trouble reaching his higher register. He also complained that his voice seemed to lose strength after 15–20 minutes of talking, which had never happened to him before. His diet and lifestyle consisted of occasional cigarette smoking and drinking alcohol socially. "I only have a few cigarettes when I'm drinking alcohol, and that only happens when I go out at night to noisy places in the City. I guess I have to speak very loudly to be heard at those places, but that only happens once or twice a week, typically on weekend nights." Albert also mentioned that he speaks on his cell phone outdoors as he's walking from appointment to appointment.

Albert drank two cups of coffee every morning, one or two Diet Cokes a day, and an occasional breath mint to drown out the tobacco smell. He never had experienced heartburn, had no history of ulcer disease, no abdominal pain or nausea, and never had an examination of his esophagus.

INITIAL EXAMINATION FINDINGS

I performed a head and neck physical examination on Albert and it was normal. A Strobe exam of the larynx was done and showed the vocal folds to be swollen and slightly red. This swollen puffy condition was preventing the vocal folds from vibrating normally.

EXPLANATION OF FINDINGS TO THE PATIENT

In order to produce consistent and reliable sounds when talking, the vocal folds must be able to vibrate normally. When the vocal folds are swollen, for any reason, be it from a cold, yelling or screaming, and/or acid reflux injury, they will not be able to vibrate normally. Think of acid-injured vocal folds as vocal folds trying to vibrate not in air, but in thick maple syrup instead. Vocal folds should be vibrating smoothly and rapidly, like a hummingbird's wings, not in slow motion. The main culprit here is lifestyle. Smoking on top of drinking alcohol while going out to noisy places requiring Albert to speak loudly to be heard, was bad upon worse upon terrible. It's what I call the professional voice-destruction "triple play"—smoking, drinking, and yelling.

TREATMENT PLAN

The single most important part of Albert's treatment was to stop smoking cigarettes. Smoking and professional voice use are simply not compatible. Aside from the cancer-causing effects of cigarettes, everyone who smokes has acid reflux by the very nature of the physiological effects of nicotine. Nicotine loosens the LES and it stimulates pepsin receptors in the throat.

Nicotine also has a direct effect on vocal folds by causing a specific swelling of the vocal fold tissues called Reinke's (Ren-KEY's) space edema. Reinke's space is an area of the vocal fold lining that swells in response to injury. In addition to the chemical trauma of nicotine, Albert never gave his vocal folds a chance to heal by using his voice loudly at night a few times a week.

I recommended that Albert see a speech language pathologist for specialized voice therapy to relax his throat muscles that had been overused in order to compensate for his swollen vocal folds. I also put Albert on the Acid Watcher® Diet and started him on a daily PPI to help transition his healing process. I asked him to return to my office in six weeks for both an examination of his larynx and an examination of his esophagus with a TNE.

FOLLOW UP #1

Albert took my recommendations seriously and his voice fatigue began to resolve itself along with his regaining more power in his voice. He not only stopped smoking, but he eliminated alcohol and cut out all soda. He still drank a single cup of coffee every morning. He was actively undergoing speech therapy and his vocal range started to return to his normal baseline. A TNE was performed, and on the way into his esophagus, I saw that the vocal fold swelling was diminished. The esophageal exam was notable for some irregularity of the bottom portion of the esophagus at the point where the esophageal lining ended and the stomach lining began. This is called an "irregular Z-line" which is commonly seen with esophageal inflammation from acid reflux injury. The Z-line is where the esophagus ends and the stomach begins. This area is generally a smooth, flat transition zone. "Irregular" means that there are peaks and valleys in this line, like mountain peaks, which signifies inflammation, typically from acid reflux. Albert's Z-line was biopsied.

Because of the esophageal inflammation found, I continued Albert on his PPI medication. I asked him to return in three months, pending the results of the esophageal biopsies.

FOLLOW UP # 2

Albert returned to my office three months later with his voice nearly back to normal. The esophageal biopsies from the TNE showed chronic inflammation due to acid reflux disease but no Barrett. His repeat laryngeal exam showed the vocal folds to be even less swollen, so I stopped the PPI medication and substituted it for a weaker antacid medication called Pepcid (famotidine), to be taken at breakfast and dinner. I emphasized the importance of staying off tobacco and limiting caffeine intake.

Before Albert left the office, I told him that I was thrilled with how seriously he took his acid reflux disease treatment, but cautioned him about falling back on bad habits.

It's unfortunate, but about 30% of my patients start off strong with strict adherence to the Acid Watcher® Diet. However, when their symptoms begin to resolve, whether from Throatburn Reflux or Heartburn Reflux, they resume drinking alcohol, eating late at night, pouring on the spicy sauce, and generally stop taking care of themselves. Needless to say, when that happens, their symptoms come back, often times worse than before, and they need to start treatment all over again.

Smoking, even a single cigarette, is not compatible with having a reliable professional voice. It not only increases one's risk for cancer of the larynx, throat, and esophagus, but *100% of smokers have acid reflux disease*. Nicotine not only stimulates pepsin receptors in the throat, but it also loosens the LES, thereby predisposing people to acid reflux regurgitation.

> ◢ **Take-out Corner**
>
> Smoking on top of drinking, while going out to noisy places, requiring one to speak loudly to be heard, is like heaping bad upon worse upon terrible. It's what I call the professional voice-destruction "triple play"—smoking, drinking and yelling.

Hoarseness: Case #4

INITIAL PATIENT PRESENTATION

Jack was a 48-year-old business consultant who was complaining of having hoarseness for six months.

PATIENT HISTORY/COMPLAINTS

Jack said his hoarseness began about one month after having his gall bladder removed under general anesthesia, about seven months prior. Jack used his voice a great deal professionally. He drank two to three cans of iced tea daily and at night had wine with dinner. He had business dinners at least twice a week which typically extended the evening until close to midnight. On those nights, his cocktail of choice was vodka combined with a heavily caffeinated energy drink. By the time he got home from his business dinners he was so exhausted that he "hit the sack" as soon as he got home. Every morning, Jack jump-started his day with two large cups of iced coffee followed by a single glass of fresh squeezed grapefruit juice. He enjoyed fried foods and balsamic vinegar in his salad dressing on his daily tomato salad with lunch. Jack had smoked cigarettes but only while in college and he never had any stomach ulcer, abdominal pain, or nausea. He never had heartburn.

INITIAL EXAMINATION FINDINGS

Jack's head and neck exam was normal. A Strobe exam of his larynx was performed which showed a large mass on the back end of his left vocal fold (see Figure A.1). In addition, the back of his larynx was quite swollen.

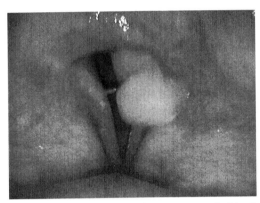

Figure A.1 Large acid reflux induced granuloma, represented by the pale, two-lobed mass on the left side of the airway.

EXPLANATION OF FINDINGS TO THE PATIENT

The most likely explanation for Jack's findings was that the breathing tube, used to control his airway during his gallbladder surgery, slightly traumatized the back of his larynx. Since his larynx was probably already quite swollen from his prodigious high-acid diet (coffee, iced tea, alcohol, citrus, vinegar, fries, etc.), he was prime to have a problem from the breathing tube being inserted into his windpipe during general anesthesia. Even the slightest bit of trauma from the breathing tube would allow all the acid being poured down his throat to severely irritate the back portion of the larynx, which is the area closest to the beginning of the esophagus. Hence, a huge granuloma ensued. A granuloma is a benign tumor which represents the body's response to inflammation. Untreated, this granuloma might have continued to grow, not only causing hoarseness, but it also could have ultimately caused Jack's airway to narrow so much that his breathing would have become impaired.

TREATMENT PLAN

Jack's treatment consisted of getting on the Acid Watcher® Diet, which included cutting out iced coffee, iced tea, alcohol, energy drinks, fried food, and vinegar. In addition, he was advised to try to start his business dinners earlier than usual. I also prescribed a PPI twice a day, to be taken 30–60 minutes before breakfast and dinner. Given Jack's hoarseness symptoms, plus his voracious acidic meals and large granuloma, I was concerned about his esophagus, so I asked him to return to my office in six weeks not only to re-examine his larynx, but also to have a TNE.

FOLLOW UP #1

Six weeks later, Jack's voice was somewhat improved, though nowhere near his baseline voice strength. I was eager to see how his granuloma was doing, so on the way to examining Jack's esophagus during the TNE, I had Jack inhale and exhale slowly while hovering over the larynx. The granuloma was still there, though it had begun to shrink (see Figure A. 2). From the larynx, I then entered the esophagus which showed a moderate amount of inflammation for almost its entire length. There was no ulceration. As I approached the bottom portion of the esophagus, near where the stomach begins, I saw that Jack had an irregular Z-line consistent with the inflammation caused by his long standing acidic diet. There was no evidence of Barrett esophagus. The TNE scope was then passed into the top of the stomach which showed a small hiatal hernia. I performed biopsies of the inflamed areas of the esophagus. Because the granuloma was still there, and because of the esophageal inflammation, I asked Jack to continue the Sustainable Phase of the Acid Watcher® Diet, to continue the twice daily PPI, and to return in six more weeks.

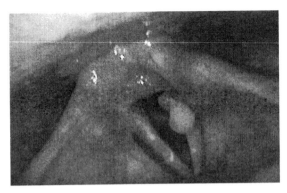

Figure A.2 Left vocal fold granuloma, appears to be shrinking in size compared with exam from six weeks earlier (Figure A.1).

FOLLOW UP #2

Six weeks later on the second follow up exam, Jack's voice was much better, though he still noticed a bit of voice fatigue towards the end of the day. The esophageal biopsies showed inflammation but no Barrett. He was following the Sustainable Phase of the Acid Watcher® Diet and was meticulous about his PPI intake. His laryngeal exam showed the left sided granuloma to be markedly improved (see Figure A.3). I asked Jack to continue the Sustainable Phase of the Acid Watcher® Diet. Because the mass was shrinking, I told him to stop the evening PPI and asked him to return to my office in three months.

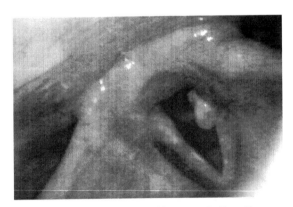

Figure A.3 Left vocal fold granuloma, shrinking even further, three months after treatment began.

FOLLOW UP #3

Three months later, Jack returned for his third follow-up exam. Now Jack's voice was back to his baseline normal state. He was quite compliant with the Sustainable Phase of the Acid Watcher® Diet and was on the morning PPI. His laryngeal exam now showed that the left sided granuloma had disappeared (see Figure A.4). I asked Jack to continue the Sustainable Phase of the Acid Watcher® Diet and to stop his PPI. I also advised taking 150 mg of ranitidine at bedtime.

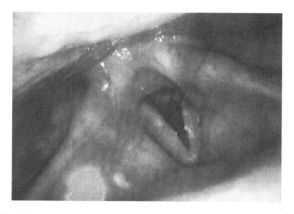

Figure A.4 Resolution of left vocal fold granuloma. Compare to Figures A.1, 2, and 3.

TAKE HOME MESSAGE

Any type of throat trauma, from being intubated during a surgical procedure under general anesthesia, to screaming loudly, can injure the larynx, predisposing it to further injury from underlying acid reflux disease. The combination of trauma and acid reflux can result in the formation of benign, inflammatory masses of the vocal folds, almost always located at the posterior, or back portion of the larynx, right near the esophageal inlet, the area where the esophagus begins. Almost always, treatment of the granuloma

> ◤**Take-out Corner**
>
> Any type of throat trauma, from being intubated during a surgical procedure under general anesthesia, to screaming loudly, can injure the larynx, predisposing it to further injury from underlying acid reflux disease.

with non-surgical means, such as a low-acid diet and antacid medications, can result in resolution of the granuloma without any type of surgical intervention. Of course, if the presumed inflammatory mass is not shrinking in size, then a biopsy should be performed to ensure that the mass is truly a benign process.

Cough: Case #1

INITIAL PATIENT PRESENTATION

Nadia, a 36-year-old saleswoman, was complaining of having a persistent cough for over a year.

PATIENT HISTORY/COMPLAINTS

Nadia had to travel on a plane two to three times a month for work. Her cough began one year prior, while travelling to Jamaica for vacation. The cough came and went, daytime and nighttime, and she said that perfumes, odors, and talking did not trigger the cough. In addition to coughing, she occasionally felt thick mucus in her throat in the morning when she woke up, which she had trouble clearing out completely.

On the mornings when she had the throat clearing problem, she thought her voice was slightly raspy, but by the time she had her morning coffee and got to her first sales call, her hoarseness seemed to go away. Her diet consisted of either fried fish (snapper, catfish) or fried chicken, generally seasoned with vinegar, chives, onion and garlic, which she ate three to four times a week. Nadia drank an occasional rum and Coke, rarely had chocolate, and did not eat mint. She worked out twice a week and was a lifetime non-smoker. She had no history of stomach ulcer disease, abdominal pain, or nausea. She never had an upper GI endoscopy.

Extensive workup of her cough, prior to seeing me, included allergy testing which showed she was allergic to dust, cockroaches, and cats. No food allergies were detected. Her chest X-ray was negative and she was not taking any medication. Her primary physician treated Nadia with a PPI called Prilosec (omeprazole) which she stopped after three weeks because her cough did not improve.

INITIAL EXAMINATION FINDINGS

To examine Nadia, I performed a TFL and saw that her vocal folds were swollen, but without redness. The vocal folds were opening and closing symmetrically, thereby indicating no sign of nerve injury. The back part of her larynx, the area just in front of where the esophagus begins, was also swollen. The spaces between the true vocal folds and the tissue above the true vocal folds, known as the false vocal folds, were obliterated and there was swelling of the tissues underneath the true vocal folds. There was a little bit of mucus on the back part of the larynx. Overall, Nadia had a swollen, puffy larynx.

EXPLANATION OF FINDINGS TO THE PATIENT

The swelling of the entire larynx, especially the vocal folds, was the likely cause of Nadia's cough. In particular, Nadia's highly acidic diet, specifically, fried chicken or fish three to four times a week, dressed with vinegar (pH 2-3) with onion and garlic (potent looseners of the LES), are likely the source of her acid reflux disease.

TREATMENT PLAN

Nadia's treatment plan consisted of a two-pronged approach—diet and medication. She was placed on the Acid Watcher® Diet, plus medical treatment, initially with a PPI. I urged Nadia to continue the low-acid diet and the medication for at least a three-month period and would re-examine her larynx at six weeks. Also at the next visit I would perform a TNE.

FOLLOW UP #1

Nadia returned 10 weeks later with her cough nearly resolved. I performed a TNE which showed the vocal folds to be less swollen and a reduction in the swelling of the back portion of the larynx near the esophageal inlet (see Chapter 2, Figure 2.1). It also revealed a small hiatal hernia and mild esophageal inflammation.

Given Nadia's improvement, both symptom-wise and the results from the TNE, I stopped the PPI and began a less strong, but still potent, antacid medication, Zantac (ranitidine), to be taken at breakfast and dinner. The instructions I gave her was to continue adherence to the Acid Watcher® Diet and to come back to be reevaluated in three months.

FOLLOW UP #2

Three months later, Nadia returned for her second follow up visit. She had noticed that the cough occurred only when she would diverge from the Acid Watcher® Diet by eating foods such as deep fried fish and chicken, and vinegar-based seasonings (her old standbys). After she had noticed this, Nadia became more diligent in following my diet recommendations and began baking and grilling her chicken and fish, as well as avoiding the heavy, acidic seasonings that she had grown accustomed to. Because of her improvement, I was able to stop her antacid medications entirely.

TAKE HOME MESSAGES

In a non-smoker with chronic cough who has a normal chest X-ray and no sinus disease or allergies, acid reflux disease must be considered as the primary cause of the cough. What the patient eats on a routine basis often plays a pivotal role in the development of acid reflux and its symptoms, in this case, chronic cough. Nadia frequently consumed fried foods, seasoned with substances that were either directly acidic (such as vinegar), or seasoned with foods that loosen the LES (such as onion and garlic). Her diet contributed to her acid reflux induced vocal fold swelling, and therefore, her cough.

Another important "take home message" is that many patients stop their antacid medication too quickly if they don't experience almost immediate relief of their symptoms. In Nadia's case, she stopped her antacid medication after three weeks because her cough did not resolve itself. In addition, she continued to consume highly acidic foods. However, if you think about it for a moment, an injury to the body caused by years and years of an unhealthy lifestyle and a highly acidic diet will not resolve itself in a few weeks. A general rule of thumb in treating Throatburn Reflux is that at six weeks of antacid medication use and low-acid eating, only 25% of patients improve, whereas at 12 weeks of antacid medication and proper diet, 75% of patients improve. Therefore, I let my patients know that it may take three months or longer for their throat symptoms related to acid reflux to resolve.

Cough: Case #2

INITIAL PATIENT PRESENTATION

Gene, a 66-year-old general contractor, had a chronic cough for the past two years.

PATIENT HISTORY/COMPLAINTS

Gene, an expert in building renovation and light construction, started coughing around the time he supervised a condominium demolition two years ago. The cough was dry, periodic, and occurred at any time of the day or night. There was nothing in particular that triggered his cough. Gene also has occasional throat clearing and a post nasal drip sensation. He did report occasional abdominal pain without nausea, but said he did not suffer from heartburn, regurgitation, difficulty swallowing, hoarseness, frequent throat clearing, or weight loss. Gene had a history of seasonal allergies, though it had been years since he took any allergy medication. His primary doctor placed him on antihistamines and nasal steroid sprays thinking allergies were the source of his cough, but the cough persisted.

He was then sent to a lung specialist who listened to Gene's chest, which was clear, obtained a chest X-ray which was negative, and ordered pulmonary function tests. The pulmonary tests were all negative. Gene was given some asthma medicine, which after a few weeks of use did not seem to help. He had a cocktail every night, usually a vodka martini, and red wine with dinner. Because of his schedule, Gene often didn't start dinner until 9–10 PM. He never smoked and did not eat mint or chocolate, and he rarely ate fried food.

INITIAL EXAMINATION FINDINGS

I performed a TFL on Gene and saw that his vocal folds and entire larynx were swollen and a bit red. There was no evidence of vocal fold weakness or abnormal vocal fold movement. There was thick post nasal drip and mucus which appeared to be stuck to portions of his throat.

EXPLANATION OF FINDINGS TO THE PATIENT

I explained to Gene that his cough was most likely due to his swollen larynx as a result of his nightly alcohol intake which was causing acid to reflux up into his throat area, a disease called Throatburn Reflux. Since Gene never complained of heartburn, he was mystified that he could possibly have acid reflux. I explained that he was likely numb in his esophagus from long standing acid injury from the chronic use of alcohol.

TREATMENT PLAN

I strongly encouraged Gene to stop drinking alcohol for at least the following four weeks. I also placed Gene on the Acid Watcher® Diet as well as PPI medication. In addition, I wanted Gene to have an upper GI endoscopy to rule out esophageal disease, as well as anything going on in his stomach. I arranged a six week follow-up appointment for Gene.

FOLLOW UP #1

Gene returned six weeks later with persistent cough. He was compliant with the antacid medication, stopped the wine, but wasn't able to give up his nightly vodka cocktail. I asked for the results of his upper endoscopy but he said the GI doctor told him he didn't need one right away because he didn't have any heartburn.

I explained to Gene my concern about persistent throat symptoms without an examination of his esophagus. I mentioned that we could do an endoscopic exam of his esophagus without using sedation called TNE. The original reason I wanted an upper GI endoscopy was because of Gene's vague abdominal discomfort, since the TNE doesn't examine the stomach well. Nevertheless, I then performed a TNE on Gene which revealed a "finger-like" projection of salmon-colored tissue coming up from his stomach and extending up into his esophagus. I biopsied this area, and the pathology report came back as Barrett esophagus which increases one's risk for developing esophageal adenocarcinoma.

I told Gene that because of the Barrett diagnosis, he would need to be followed on a regular basis by his GI physician with periodic upper endoscopies. In the meantime, I prescribed for Gene PPI medication once a day in the morning and strongly recommended that he follow the Acid Watcher® Diet without exception, which meant stopping *all* alcohol.

FOLLOW UP #2

Gene returned to my office three months later with his cough almost completely resolved. He did have an upper GI endoscopy (also known as an EsophagoGastroDuodenoscopy (EGD) with a different GI doctor which not only confirmed Barrett esophagus, but also showed a stomach ulcer. His PPI medication was subsequently increased to twice daily. Gene was now finally convinced to stop alcohol completely.

TAKE HOME MESSAGE

Nightly alcohol use can cause enough acid injury to the esophagus to result in severe esophageal inflammation, even possibly Barrett esophagus. It can also cause chronic cough. If you have persistent throatburn symptoms, whether or not you also have heartburn, your esophagus should be examined (see TIDE, Chapter 5).

Throat Clearing: Case #1

INITIAL PATIENT PRESENTATION

Walter, a 70-year-old accountant, complained of having eight years of constant throat clearing which began after a bout of "laryngitis."

PATIENT HISTORY/COMPLAINTS

By way of greeting, my new patient Walter said to me, "Doctor, I got so much phlegm in my throat. I'm sick of the mucus in my throat. I make too much mucus. Can you get rid of the mucus? I know it's my post nasal drip, I've had this drip for many years, but it's getting worse as I'm getting older!" I asked Walter if he ever had heartburn and he told me that he'd never had it. Because of slightly abnormal blood tests found by his primary care doctor, Walter had an upper GI endoscopy the previous year which showed a small hiatal hernia and some mild inflammation of his stomach. His GI doctor placed him on Nexium, which Walter took for two weeks but then stopped. According to Walter, "It wasn't working."

He had had evaluations by lung doctors, allergists, and other ENT doctors and was given antihistamines, decongestants, nasal steroid sprays, and asthma medication, none of which helped. He had a neurology consultation to make sure he didn't have any hidden chronic neurological diseases like Lou Gehrig's Disease (Amyotrophic Lateral Sclerosis—ALS), Parkinson's disease, or myasthenia gravis. The neurology consult was negative. He was even told he should see a psychiatrist because after all these negative tests perhaps this was "all in his head."

Walter was very frustrated and further complained that his co-workers could hear him walking down the hall, constantly clearing his throat, ready to hock up his phlegm.

Diet and lifestyle-wise, he was a lifetime non-smoker, had nightly one to two glasses of either red or white wine, and loved tomato sauce, especially with pasta which he had twice a week. For breakfast, he always had a glass of orange juice, no more than one cup of coffee daily, no mint, rarely ate fried foods, and drank soda only when he was watching a movie, which was about once a week.

INITIAL EXAMINATION FINDINGS

Walter had a normal head and neck physical examination. Because of Walter's complaints of excess throat phlegm suggesting a swallowing problem, I then performed a FEESST (Flexible Endoscopic Evaluation of Swallowing with Sensory Testing, see Chapter 3) on Walter and detected four abnormal findings. The first was that his larynx was quite swollen. Even more dramatic, a second finding was that during the sensory testing portion of the FEESST exam, he was slightly numb on the left side of his throat compared to his right side. Normally, the sensory test should show the right and left sides of the throat to have equal sensitivities. The third abnormal result was that, when the FEESST camera was in his throat observing his vocal fold movement, his entire larynx twisted to one side when he was asked to say a five second long "eeeeeeeee" followed by a short sniff. (This is a standard physiological prompt that allows the physician to see certain vocal fold movements clearly). The fourth abnormal finding was that saliva was building up on the left side of his larynx.

EXPLANATION OF FINDINGS TO THE PATIENT

The swelling in the back of the larynx, near where the esophagus begins, strongly suggests acid reflux injury to Walter's vocal folds. The other three abnormalities indicate that Walter had a nerve injury to the particular nerve that provides movement and sensation to the left vocal fold.

How can these abnormalities cause frequent throat clearing? This happens in two ways. Please take a look once again at Figures 2.1 and 2.2 of Chapter 2, showing the normal and acid injured larynx. In an acid injured larynx, the back portion of the larynx will often be swollen. As a result, the one to two liters a day of mucus that is normally produced from the nose and sinuses will actually sit on the swollen larynx, just like a shelf holding up books. Except now the larynx is the shelf holding up a library amount of mucus and phlegm.

In Walter's situation, what made things much worse was that his left vocal fold was partially paralyzed. When the vocal fold nerve is injured, either partially or completely, the UES (upper esophageal sphincter, explained in depth in Chapter 2) cannot relax normally. In fact, the nerve that sends a message to the UES to relax during swallowing is the same nerve that provides motor and sensory information to the larynx. It's called the **vagus nerve**. So it is actually typical for a vocal fold nerve injury to have a "side effect" of frequent throat clearing. In fact, almost any time a patient comes in to see me with a chief complaint of relentless, frequent throat clearing, I am always on the lookout for subtle nerve injury, especially after they have seen multiple specialists over a long period of time.

Frequently, in patients presenting with throat complaints, whether it's Throatburn Reflux or Heartburn Reflux, acid reflux disease should be entertained as a diagnosis and then treated. However, if the nerve injury component is not recognized, then the throat clearing symptom can persist.

TREATMENT PLAN

Once a diagnosis of a nerve injury is made, what does one do? Fortunately, there exists an isometric head and neck exercise called Shaker exercises (pronounced Shah-kehr) that can be administered to loosen the tight, or non-relaxing, UES muscles. While there are several ways to loosen a tight or poorly relaxing UES, Shaker exercises are the safest method to apply in this type of situation.

What you essentially do is lie down on your back with a pillow behind your head. You then lift your head and look at your feet, holding your head up for five seconds, then putting your head back down on the pillow. Each subsequent day your head is held up for five more seconds until, after a two to three week period, you can hold your head up for one minute, then rest for one minute and repeat two more times. Typically, six weeks of Shaker exercises can loosen the tight UES and the frequent throat clearing sensation will often resolve.

In Walter's situation, because his nerve injury was newly diagnosed, I had to make sure there was no tumor in his neck or chest pressing on the nerve that moves the vocal folds. I consequently ordered an MRI of his neck and a CT scan of his chest. I also put Walter on the Acid Watcher® Diet and placed him back on his antacid medication.

FOLLOW UP

Eight weeks later, Walter returned to my office with his throat clearing much improved. He was still performing the Shaker exercises. Fortunately, his CT scan and MRI were both negative. Examination of his larynx showed persistent subtle weakness of the left vocal fold. However, the saliva that had been pooling on the left side of his larynx had resolved. He was advised to continue his antacid medications as well as the Acid Watcher® Diet.

TAKE HOME MESSAGE

Persistent throat symptoms after maximum treatment of acid induced laryngeal injury should point one towards a *nerve* injury to be contributing to the patient's symptoms. Invariably, nerve injuries of the larynx exacerbate the effects of acid induced laryngeal injury. In general, this case history underscores the following basic tenet of medicine: Without a proper diagnosis, it is very difficult to *properly* treat a patient.

Throat Clearing: Case #2

INITIAL PATIENT PRESENTATION

Roger, a 74-year-old retiree, was complaining of worsening throat clearing for the last six months.

PATIENT HISTORY/COMPLAINTS

Roger had a history of seasonal allergies for decades, so when he initially started clearing his throat, he first went to his primary physician to have his antihistamine medications and nasal steroid sprays adjusted. However, his throat clearing not only persisted but got worse. In the past month, before coming in to see me, Roger had to carry around a small box of tissues because he was spitting up his phlegm with greater frequency.

He had a normal upper GI endoscopy three years earlier because he was having some abdominal discomfort which turned out to be gall bladder disease. His gall bladder problem ended up being controlled without surgery. Diet and lifestyle-wise, Roger stopped smoking cigarettes in the 1960s, drank one cup of coffee per day, and had nightly wine with dinner, usually eaten around 6:30 PM. He occasionally ate chocolate and mint, not much fried foods, and no soda or seltzer. Roger didn't have any heartburn complaints.

INITIAL EXAMINATION FINDINGS

Roger's head and neck exam was notable for an abnormal appearance of his tongue surface. When asked to open his mouth, which is a routine part of every head and neck examination I perform, I noticed that the tongue had subtle wiggling of its surface, like a worm was moving just underneath the surface of the tongue. When he stuck his tongue out, the wiggling persisted. The name for this type of involuntary tongue wiggling is tongue fasciculations (fah-sick-u-lay-shins). He was able to move his tongue side to side but his tongue movement seemed a bit sluggish. I performed a FEESST exam on Roger because I was concerned that his throat clearing was due to some alteration in his swallowing mechanism. When I passed the FEESST camera into Roger's throat, there was build-up of secretions near his larynx. He had bilateral sensory deficits that were symmetric and when he swallowed there was residual food in the areas by his vocal folds. There was a moderate amount of swelling in the back of his larynx.

EXPLANATION OF FINDINGS TO THE PATIENT

The tongue wiggling may indicate that Roger's tongue muscles were weak. The persistent mucus secretions in Roger's throat, which is the reason he had the frequent throat clearing complaint, were caused by two different reasons. The first was due to the combination of the tongue fasciculations along with the fact that his larynx did not elevate normally during his swallow. These findings meant that the muscles of swallowing (tongue and throat) were likely neurologically impaired and thus slightly denervated, or nerve-injured, causing the muscles to not move well.

The second reason for the secretions was because of acid reflux, which caused swelling of the back of the larynx. As previously described in other case histories, posterior laryngeal swelling acts like a shelf, upon which secretions can build up.

TREATMENT PLAN

To treat his laryngeal swelling, Roger was placed on the Acid Watcher® Diet and antacid medications. However, the key next step was to have Roger see a neurologist to make sure there was no chronic neurodegenerative process taking place.

FOLLOW UP

Six weeks later, Roger returned to my office with his throat clearing slightly improved. He saw the neurologist who, after extensive testing, felt there was some type of chronic nerve injury taking place called a Parkinson-like syndrome. He placed Roger on medications to address his underlying neurological disease.

TAKE HOME MESSAGE

While constant throat clearing is often due to untreated or insufficiently treated acid reflux disease, it may also be a consequence of impaired movement of throat and tongue muscles. While chronic neurological disease is somewhat unusual, it must be in the range of diagnostic possibilities when such complaints are being brought to a physician's attention. If muscle injury is suspected, the acid reflux component should be treated, but that's not all that should be done. A neurology consultation is a very important part of the diagnostic workup under these types of circumstances.

Difficulty Swallowing (Dysphagia): Case #1

INITIAL PATIENT PRESENTATION

Annabel, a 24-year-old public relations account executive, came into my office complaining of difficulty swallowing pills for the past year.

PATIENT HISTORY/COMPLAINTS

In addition to her difficulty in swallowing pills, Annabel also noted a lump-like sensation in her throat for the last year. Furthermore, for the past three months, she felt increasingly scared to eat solid food and as a result had lost five pounds during this time period. She pointed to her Adam's apple to indicate the precise area where food seemed to be held up. She never had any imaging (MRI or CT scan) studies. She had no heartburn complaints and was a lifetime non-smoker.

Since her second year of college she started her day with two skim milk cappuccinos and a glass of orange juice for breakfast. Her job required attending late night events two to three nights a week so on those nights she didn't eat dinner until 10 PM.

INITIAL EXAMINATION FINDINGS

A FEESST was performed which showed bilateral symmetric laryngeal sensory deficits and severe swelling of the back portion of her vocal fold region. While I didn't see food sitting on the back of her throat after she swallowed, thick throat mucus or phlegm did sit on the back of the larynx after every swallow.

EXPLANATION OF FINDINGS TO THE PATIENT

Annabel's difficulty in swallowing and the lump-like sensation in her throat were due to Throatburn Reflux which caused rather significant swelling of her throat tissues. The primary culprits of her Throatburn Reflux were the cappuccino-orange juice duo and the late night meals several times per week.

TREATMENT PLAN

I explained to Annabel that, in general, her type of vocal fold swelling was reversible provided that she adjust her diet and lifestyle and take antacid medication. I recommended that she begin the Acid Watcher® Diet, limit late night eating, and begin a morning PPI. In addition, I wanted her to obtain an X-ray test of the esophagus called a Barium Swallow, or esophagram, to make sure there was no blockage anywhere in her esophagus.

FOLLOW UP

During a follow-up examination eight weeks later, Annabel reported lessening of the lump-like sensation in her throat but it was still an issue for her. The esophagram showed nothing abnormal. Her coffee/orange juice breakfast was replaced with Acid Watcher® Diet breakfasts. The late night eating was unavoidable because of her work responsibilities.

A physical exam of Annabel showed the back of her larynx to be much less swollen. I advised her to continue the Acid Watcher® Diet as strictly as possible, and to continue her antacid medication. It was reiterated to her that her late night eating was going to slow the healing of the swelling of the back of her larynx.

TAKE HOME MESSAGE

One of the most common causes of difficulty swallowing in a young, otherwise healthy individual is swelling of the back of the larynx due to acid reflux disease.

Difficulty Swallowing (Dysphagia): Case #2

INITIAL PATIENT PRESENTATION

Michael, a 69-year-old man, was complaining of difficulty swallowing for one year after suffering from a stroke.

PATIENT HISTORY/COMPLAINTS

Michael had a stroke a year ago which resulted in temporary weakness of his right arm and leg. He also noticed that it was more difficult for him to swallow solid foods after the stroke. He told this to his neurologist, who sent Michael to have an X-ray test of swallowing performed in the presence of a speech language pathologist, called a Modified Barium Swallow (MBS). The MBS showed that there was some impairment of elevation of the throat muscles and some mild weakness of the throat muscles, but no aspiration (choking) on solid or liquid food. He was advised to eat softer foods of almost a puréed consistency and to eat slowly. One year later, Michael was tired of puréeing his food so he was referred to me to evaluate his swallowing mechanism.

He revealed that he had no episodes of pneumonia since his stroke and his weight was stable. Diet and lifestyle details consisted of Michael having quit cigarette smoking in the 1980s. He had a daily morning cup of coffee, occasional wine with dinner, several iced teas a day, and spicy foods three to four times per week.

INITIAL EXAMINATION FINDINGS

A FEESST exam was performed which showed impairment of strength of his throat muscles as well as a large amount of swelling at the back part of the larynx with thick mucus stuck in that area.

EXPLANATION OF FINDINGS TO THE PATIENT

Michael had two causes for his swallowing problems. One was a neurological problem as a result of his stroke, resulting in weakness of his pharyngeal, or throat muscles. The other source was acid reflux causing swelling of his larynx, adding a mechanical problem (swelling of the throat) to his existing neurological problem.

TREATMENT PLAN

To treat both of these causes, I asked Michael to see a speech language pathologist specializing in isometric exercises to improve swallowing. I also placed him on the Acid Watcher® Diet and PPIs, and asked him to come back to see me in three months.

FOLLOW UP

Three months later Michael returned with less difficulty swallowing and no episodes of aspiration pneumonia. His weight was stable. He did work with a speech pathologist who helped him with his swallowing mechanics. He was continuing on the Acid Watcher® Diet and taking his antacid medications. A repeat FEESST exam showed much less mucus in the back of his larynx and less overall swelling of his larynx as well. He was advised to continue the swallowing therapy exercises on his own and to continue the Acid Watcher® Diet along with his PPIs.

TAKE HOME MESSAGE

Throatburn Reflux can worsen any type of swallowing problem, whether it be after a stroke or in someone with neurological disease. Therefore, addressing laryngeal (throat) swelling from Throatburn Reflux can generally improve swallowing problems.

Hoarseness and Regurgitation Case

INITIAL PATIENT PRESENTATION

Dominik, a 38-year-old male professional singer, was complaining that for the past six months he was unable to reach the upper register of his voice while singing.

PATIENT HISTORY/COMPLAINTS

Dominik mentioned that for the past six months he suffered from occasional regurgitation of food all the way into his mouth, as well as a lump-like sensation in his throat after a meal. I asked him if he would ever lie down shortly after eating a meal and he responded, "Doctor, I usually eat in bed lying down and often fall asleep right after eating!" Inquiring about his lifestyle habits, Dominik reported that he had an occasional cigarette and drank alcohol two to three times per week, usually when going out with friends. He had two cups of coffee per day, liked chocolate, didn't eat mint, occasional ate fried food, and had daily grapefruit juice after his coffee. He frequently ate tomato, onion, and garlic, typically in the form of pizza, at least once a week. He did not have any heartburn.

INITIAL EXAMINATION FINDINGS

Because of my concern that something might be obstructing Dominik's throat or esophagus, I performed a TNE on him during his initial visit. During the TNE, I observed that the back portion of his larynx, at the location where the esophagus starts, was very swollen. In fact, immediately upon entering his esophagus, I noticed that the entire length of it was highly inflamed. In addition, at the bottom of the esophagus, I identified a small hiatal hernia. While at the bottom (distal) portion of the esophagus, I also performed biopsies.

EXPLANATION OF FINDINGS TO THE PATIENT

I explained to Dominik that he had Throatburn Reflux. In addition, while his TNE showed that he had no obstruction anywhere in his esophagus, he did have severe acid injury to his larynx and esophagus.

TREATMENT PLAN

I recommended that he immediately start on the Acid Watcher® Diet and twice daily PPI. I emphasized to Dominik the importance of following the Acid Watcher® Diet non-negotiables (see Chapter 8), which includes waiting at least three hours after eating before lying down, no cigarettes, and no alcohol. Additionally, I asked him to return in six to eight weeks for a follow-up exam.

FOLLOW UP

Dominik returned to my office about two months later, saying that his voice had improved somewhat, and that he had much less regurgitation. His esophageal biopsies showed chronic inflammation, without Barrett. He completely stopped eating in a near lying down position, stopped the social smoking, and eliminated alcohol. However, he was not able to eliminate coffee and pizza completely. He only "cut it down." I reminded him that he wasn't being fully compliant with the Acid Watcher® Diet and that's why his voice was not back to its full shape. I advised Dominik to continue staying upright after meals and to be more adherent to the Acid Watcher® Diet if he wanted to make a full recovery and be able to once again use his complete vocal range.

TAKE HOME MESSAGE

Diet and lifestyle are pivotal factors in the development of Throatburn Reflux symptoms. The good news is that the changes in the throat and vocal folds as a result of acid injury are almost always reversible.

APPENDIX B:
True Patient Stories About Vocal Cord Dysfunction (VCD)

"Therein the patient must minister to himself."

—SHAKESPEARE

As was discussed throughout the book, the most common non-lung, non-allergy cause of chronic cough is acid reflux disease. However, there is another cause of chronic cough which is often overlooked, called vocal cord dysfunction (VCD). The medical term for VCD is also known as Paradoxical Vocal Fold Movement Disorder (PVFMD).

WHAT IS VCD?

VCD, described for the first time in 1983, is a disease of unknown etiology, which means we don't know why it happens. Normally, the vocal folds are wide open during quiet breathing. With VCD, however, the vocal folds stay closed, or nearly so, for up to several seconds during quiet breathing, hence the term "**paradoxical**," where the paradox is the vocal folds shutting during quiet breathing, instead of staying open. As the vocal folds begin to move towards each other, they close the airway, thereby restricting the movement of air going into the lungs. This closing of the vocal folds may cause one to feel shortness of breath, followed by a sensation of choking, which ultimately leads to cough.

Although VCD has been described for years, it has never made it into the mainstream of public knowledge. Part of the reason no one has ever heard of this disease is that various names have been given to describe this condition that have appeared in the pulmonary, gastric, otolaryngology, speech, and psychiatric literature. Some of the names attributed to VCD are *stridor, factitious asthma,* and *irritable larynx.*

While the cause of VCD is not known, it is believed to be related to some type of problem with the Vagus nerve (the 10th cranial nerve). This is the nerve from the brain that governs most throat functions, including speech, voice, swallowing, and breathing. Therefore, anything that stimulates the throat, especially Throatburn Reflux, can produce VCD symptoms.

VCD is associated with a high incidence of both GastroEsophageal Reflux Disease (GERD), or Heartburn Reflux, and LaryngoPharyngeal Reflux (LPR), or Throatburn Reflux.

Symptoms of VCD

The most common symptom of VCD is chronic cough. That's a cough that lasts more than eight weeks. Sometimes, the VCD cough can go on for decades until a correct diagnosis is made. Generally, the cough associated with VCD is a daytime cough, typically triggered by speaking, odors, perfumes, soaps, soap powders, smoke, household cleaners, drinking and/or eating, or temperature changes. Occasionally, exercise and anxiety can trigger the cough. Other symptoms besides cough, such as throat tightness, throat spasm, choking sensation, shortness of breath, lump-like sensation in throat, difficulty swallowing, and neck tightness may also present as VCD.

Diagnosis of VCD

VCD is diagnosed in two ways. One way is during examination of the larynx with a camera, a procedure known as Transnasal Flexible Laryngoscopy (TFL, see Chapter 4). The examiner looks for the aforementioned vocal fold closing pattern during quiet breathing. Often, I have a patient say a particular sentence as a means of eliciting the vocal fold closing movement typical of VCD. For example, I like to have the patient say, "We see three green trees" and then observe vocal fold movement. What happens in a normal situation is that the vocal folds should open after a sentence is said, corresponding to the patient taking a breath. However, with VCD, the vocal folds will close, and stay closed, after a sentence is said.

The other way to make a diagnosis, besides examining the larynx with a camera, is with a form of *pulmonary function testing*, or testing of the lungs, called Spirometry. Spirometry measures the amount, or volume, and speed of air that can be inhaled and exhaled during breathing. With Spirometry, the patient breathes in (inspiration) and out (expiration) through a device called a Spirometer, and the amount and speed of air flow to and from the lungs is calculated. This measurement is called a **flow-volume loop**. A normal flow-volume loop essentially looks like a circle, with a horizontal line right through the middle of the circle (see Figure B). The upper part of the circle represents breath flow during expiration, while the bottom half represents air flow during inspiration. Normally, the upper and lower parts of the circle are somewhat equal in size. In patients with VCD, because the vocal folds are closed or narrowed during inspiration, the amount of air flow is limited, so the bottom part of the flow-volume loop circle is flattened (see Figure B).

> ### ▛ Take-out Corner
> When you are coming to your ENT doctor for investigation of your chronic cough, and you have already been to the lung doctor and had a Spirometry, please bring that Spirometry tracing to your ENT physician. That information can greatly help with making your diagnosis.

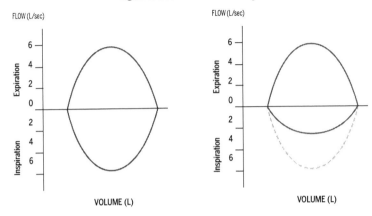

Figure B Flow-Volume loop.

There are two flow-volume loops being shown. The one on the left is normal, showing that breath flow during expiration (top portion of the curve) and inspiration (bottom portion of the curve) are symmetrical. The other flow-volume loop, the one on the right, is abnormal, showing a flattening of the inspiratory curve, classically seen in patients with vocal cord dysfunction. L/sec = Liters per second; L = Liters.

Treatment for VCD

It has been shown that over 80% of patients with VCD have either Heartburn Reflux (GERD) or Throatburn Reflux (LPR). Therefore, the treatment of VCD almost always involves two parts: treating the acid reflux disease component, and then implementing physical therapy techniques to address the abnormal closing of the vocal folds.

The acid reflux disease contribution is treated with a combination of the Acid Watcher® Diet as well as antacid medications.

The abnormal movement of the vocal folds is treated with a form of physical therapy administered by speech language pathologists called **respiratory retraining**. The important point to understand is that while acid reflux contributes to the VCD problem, treating the acid reflux disease alone will not rid the patient of their cough. At the same time, if the acid reflux component is not treated, then the respiratory retraining alone will generally not be sufficient to treat the cough.

WHAT IS RESPIRATORY RETRAINING?

Respiratory retraining is increased resistance breathing exercises, almost always administered by an experienced speech language pathologist. Respiratory retraining consists of a series of resistive breathing techniques which are designed to relax the vocal fold muscles during exhalation (breathing out) and inhalation (breathing in). While there are several methods, one that can be readily described involves instructing the patient to perform a "closed-lip sniff" as soon as the cough starts. By sniffing with lips tightly closed, a message gets instantly sent to the brain to immediately open the vocal folds. Once you sniff or inhale air through your nose, your lungs fill with air. The key maneuver is then to slowly force air out of your lungs though closed lips. It's almost as if one is whistling air out of one's lungs through pursed lips after the deep sniff or deep inhalation is performed.

During my years at the Columbia University Medical Center, I worked with one of the world's renowned speech language pathologists, Tom Murry, SLP, PhD. Dr. Murry perfected the technique of respiratory retraining and we published several scientific papers about VCD. Usually, four to five sessions of respiratory retraining are enough to modify the abnormal breathing pattern which in turn significantly reduces cough and its associated symptoms.

> ## ▼ Take-out Corner
> While acid reflux contributes to VCD, treating the acid reflux disease element alone will not rid the patient of their cough. At the same time, if the acid reflux component is not treated, then the respiratory retraining alone will generally not be sufficient to completely treat the cough.

TRUE PATIENT STORIES ABOUT VOCAL CORD DYSFUNCTION (VCD)

The following case histories illustrate the frustrations that typical patients with dysfunctional vocal folds go through before a correct diagnosis is made and proper treatment begins.

There are numerous published reports where some people have been coughing for up to 20 years, without relief, having gone through the medical diagnostic and specialty search treadmill, to no avail. Here are the stories of John, Kelly, and Ellen, who were lucky to get a proper diagnose and treatment for VCD.

VCD Case #1: John

INITIAL PATIENT PRESENTATION

John, a 43-year-old executive with an apparel company, was coughing and hoarse for the past year.

PATIENT HISTORY/COMPLAINTS

John's wife noticed that for the past year he was hoarse by the time he got home from his office. About two weeks after the hoarseness began, John began to cough during the day at work, at which point she urged him to see his family doctor to make sure he wasn't harboring some type of infection. His family doctor investigated the cough by listening to John's chest with a stethoscope and then obtaining a chest X-ray. The chest exam and X-ray were unremarkable. His doctor suggested that he take some antacid pills after dinner for a few weeks.

After several weeks, the hoarseness increased and the cough was more common throughout the day. People in his office began to ask if he had a cold. When he told his doctor that the antacid pills were not helping, his doctor suggested a visit to an ear, nose, and throat (ENT) doctor since

John had a distant history of smoking (though he had not smoked ciga-rettes in over 10 years). John drank two cups of coffee a day, a nightly vodka martini, rarely ate citrus or chocolate, and had a daily tomato salad with a vinegar-based dressing. He had no history of abdominal pain or nausea.

John went to an ENT doctor and was diagnosed with seasonal aller-gies and it was suggested that he begin allergy shots. Not comfortable with regularly scheduled allergy shots, he decided to seek a second opin-ion after a colleague at his company mentioned that I had helped her mother get rid of a cough she suffered from for many years.

INITIAL EXAMINATION FINDINGS

I examined John with Laryngeal Video Stroboscopy. He had swelling of the back portion of his larynx, and his vocal folds were swollen as well. During quiet breathing, when normally the vocal folds only move slightly with inspiration and expiration, his vocal folds came together and stayed closed for several seconds at a time. Every time I had John say the sen-tence "We see three green trees," his vocal folds stayed closed for almost six seconds.

EXPLANATION OF FINDINGS TO THE PATIENT

Because of sustained vocal fold closure during quiet breathing, as well as after saying a sentence, John was diagnosed with VCD. The VCD was a major cause of his cough. In addition, as a result of his laryngeal swelling, he was diagnosed with Throatburn Reflux. The swollen vocal folds were likely responsible for John's hoarseness.

TREATMENT PLAN

I started John on the Acid Watcher® Diet and gave him a proton pump inhibitor (PPI) two times a day. He was referred to a speech language pathologist for respiratory retraining. I asked John to return in six weeks for a TransNasal Esophagoscopy (TNE), given his longstanding Throatburn Reflux symptoms.

FOLLOW UP #1

Six weeks later, John returned to my office less hoarse with his cough essentially resolved. He underwent respiratory retraining and was fairly consistent about doing the exercises on a daily basis. John also stopped his nightly cocktail, except for Saturday night, and stopped using vinegar entirely. I performed a TNE which revealed the larynx to still be swollen in the back portion, though the vocal folds themselves were less swollen. Examination of the esophagus showed slight redness at the bottom of the esophagus, an irregular Z-line, no clinical Barrett esophagus (no obvious extension of salmon-colored stomach lining into the esophagus) with a small hiatal hernia (a portion of the stomach was above the diaphragm). Brush biopsies were taken of the irregular Z-line.

John was advised to continue the Acid Watcher® Diet, the PPIs, and the respiratory retraining exercises, and to return in another six weeks.

FOLLOW UP #2

Eight weeks later, John returned for another examination of his larynx. His hoarseness had resolved and he was no longer coughing. He stopped his respiratory retraining exercises a month previously, but he was maintaining the Sustainable Phase of the Acid Watcher® Diet.

The biopsies of his esophagus showed slight esophagitis or esophageal inflammation, with no Barrett esophagus. Follow-up Stroboscopy showed overall improvement in his laryngeal swelling. Also, his vocal folds were now closing normally, thereby indicating that his VCD was cured. The PPIs were stopped and John was placed on a less powerful antacid than the PPI class he had been taking, a Histamine-2 (H2)

Blocker called Zantac (ranitidine), which was to be taken at night before bedtime.

TAKE HOME MESSAGE

Chronic cough, which is a cough lasting for more than eight weeks, needs to be investigated by your primary doctor. If the cough persists, you should then see your ENT doctor to make sure that your larynx is examined as well. Moreover, with persistent cough, the esophagus should also be examined to rule out Barrett esophagus.

VCD Case #2: Kelly

INITIAL PATIENT PRESENTATION

Kelly, a musical theater singer and dancer, had been complaining of shortness of breath for the past five months.

PATIENT HISTORY/COMPLAINTS

Kelly came to New York City after graduating from a performing arts college and was auditioning for roles in a musical theater production off-Broadway. Five months ago, she developed shortness of breath after a cold. In addition, for the last three months, she was noticing a dry cough throughout the day, at times rather violent. Perfumes and odors seemed to trigger her shortness of breath as well as her cough. She never wheezed, but did have intermittent nasal congestion on both sides of her nose, typically during the spring allergy season. Kelly exercised regularly and could not relate her shortness of breath to exercise. She had a waitressing job at night and generally had her last meal after her shift ended around midnight. Every day for breakfast she had a single cup of coffee and a single glass of fresh-squeezed grapefruit juice. She drank alcohol socially, and was a lifetime non-smoker. Kelly saw a lung specialist (pulmonologist) who ruled out any heart or lung problems. He initially treated her for asthma and allergies yet her cough persisted. The pulmonologist then referred the patient to me for further evaluation.

INITIAL EXAMINATION FINDINGS

Kelly's head and neck examination was unremarkable. A TFL was performed which showed the vocal folds to be slightly swollen in the back portion of her larynx. During the TFL, she was prompted to say, "We see three green trees," and her vocal folds, instead of opening after the passage was said, immediately closed and stayed shut for eight seconds. This happened every time she said this passage.

EXPLANATION OF FINDINGS TO THE PATIENT

Kelly had paradoxical closure of the vocal folds after speaking, consistent with a diagnosis of VCD. The reason for her shortness of breath was the result of her vocal folds staying shut for several seconds at a time, much like repeatedly holding one's breath.

TREATMENT PLAN

Kelly was referred to a speech language pathologist for respiratory retraining. In addition, I had her begin the Acid Watcher® Diet, prescribed a PPI to be taken once a day, and asked her to return to my office in six weeks.

FOLLOW UP

Kelly returned for a follow-up visit three months later with her shortness of breath and cough entirely resolved. She was following the Acid Watcher® Diet, though occasionally had meals late at night. She continued to see a speech language pathologist for respiratory retraining and was meticulous about following the increased resistance breathing exercises.

TAKE HOME MESSAGE

When a young, healthy individual is complaining of shortness of breath, the heart and lungs should be examined first in order to rule out cardio-pulmonary disease. If the heart and lung exam is unremarkable, an allergy investigation is then indicated. If the allergy exam is not revelatory, the larynx should be examined by an ENT doctor to rule out laryngeal disease as a source of the shortness of breath.

VCD Case #3: Ellen

INITIAL PATIENT PRESENTATION

Ellen, a 59-year-old part-time bookkeeper from northern New York State, was complaining of having nine months of cough.

PATIENT HISTORY/COMPLAINTS

About one month before her cough began, Ellen had a severe cold. The cold went away but Ellen began coughing while talking on the telephone at work. The cough was also noticed while eating. Eventually, after eight months, she noticed that any time she began to talk to anyone, she would cough, sometimes excessively. Ellen had a history of seasonal allergies so she went to see her allergist, who identified an unusually strong cough after he gave her some perfume to smell. She told the allergist that she quit using perfume four to five years ago because it made her cough and sometimes wheeze. Because of the wheezing at that time, she saw two different pulmonologists, both of whom found her to have normal lungs but thought she might possibly have adult onset asthma. They treated her for asthma and told her to stay away from perfumes. The allergist could not identify specific food or environmental allergies so he referred the patient to me to evaluate her chronic cough.

INITIAL EXAMINATION FINDINGS

I obtained more information from Ellen about her lifestyle. She was a lifetime non-smoker and in otherwise good health without previous stomach ulcer, abdominal pain, or nausea. She drank a cup of coffee every morning but rarely had alcohol, chocolate, fried food, citrus, or garlic. On occasion she had tomatoes and onion with a vinaigrette dressing. She related to me that she stopped going out to eat at most restaurants because some of the food smells also triggered her cough. Her friends would often tell her not to talk while she was eating since talking brought on even stronger coughing.

I examined Ellen with Flexible Endoscopic Evaluation of Swallowing with Sensory Testing (FEESST). Her entire larynx was swollen and she had severe sensory deficits in and around the vocal folds. She was able to swallow food and liquids without difficulty. She recited a simple five word sentence at which point her vocal folds started to gradually close and then remained closed for several seconds. I wafted perfume some distance from her nose and her vocal folds suddenly closed for several seconds as well.

EXPLANATION OF FINDINGS TO THE PATIENT

Ellen had two processes going on—Throatburn Reflux as well as VCD. The swelling of her larynx was consistent with Throatburn Reflux disease. In addition, the gradual closure of the vocal folds after saying a sentence was consistent with VCD or paradoxical vocal fold motion. This vocal fold closure became more like a spasm of the vocal folds (the vocal folds suddenly slamming shut for several seconds) when she was given perfume to smell.

TREATMENT PLAN

Ellen was placed on the Acid Watcher® Diet and specifically advised to avoid vinegar, tomato, and onion. She was given two medication prescriptions, one for a daily morning PPI to be taken 30–60 minutes before breakfast and the other for ranitidine. She was also given a prescription to see a speech language pathologist for respiratory retraining. In addition, because of her chronic cough and lack of abdominal pain or nausea, I wanted her to return in six weeks for a TNE.

FOLLOW UP # 1

Ellen returned to my office six weeks later with minimal improvement with her cough. She was taking her medication and following the Acid Watcher® Diet but had yet to see the speech language pathologist, so respiratory retraining exercises had not yet begun. I performed a TNE which showed the larynx to be less swollen but the paradoxical vocal fold movement was still present. Her esophageal exam showed a single tongue-like projection of salmon-colored tissue above the Z-line which was biopsied. She also had a small hiatal hernia. The remainder of the TNE exam was negative. I asked Ellen to stay on the PPI/H2 blocker regimen and continue with the Sustainable Phase of the Acid Watcher® Diet. I re-emphasized the need for respiratory retraining and requested that she follow-up in six weeks. I explained that I would contact her with the biopsy results as soon as they were available.

FOLLOW UP # 2

Two months later, Ellen returned for a follow-up exam. The biopsies from the TNE showed inflammation of the esophagus without any Barrett. In addition to sticking with the Acid Watcher® Diet and PPI/H2 blocker combination, Ellen finally saw a speech language pathologist and started practicing the respiratory retraining exercises daily. As a result, Ellen's cough had resolved and she was now able to feel comfortable socializing with her friends. A follow-up TFL only showed some mild swelling of

the back of the larynx, otherwise the laryngeal swelling was markedly reduced and there was no further paradoxical vocal fold motion. I stopped
the PPI and asked Ellen to continue the ranitidine at bedtime, keep on
the Sustainable Phase of the Acid Watcher® Diet, and continue to practice her breathing exercises.

TAKE HOME MESSAGE

Cough from VCD will not improve with an antacid and low-acid diet
regimen alone. One must also routinely perform the respiratory retraining exercises as well, in order to obtain complete symptom relief.

VCD CASE HISTORIES SUMMARY

As we can see from the histories above, the cough from dysfunctional
vocal folds can continue unabated for years while many diagnostic and
therapeutic avenues are traversed until the correct diagnosis is made.
However, once the correct diagnosis is made, relief from the cough
usually follows.

GLOSSARY

"It's not food if it arrived through the window of your car."
—MICHAEL POLLAN

Acid Watcher® Diet (also known as **the Dr. Aviv Diet®**): A low-acid, nutritionally balanced, high fiber diet.

Allergist: A doctor who specializes in treating allergies.

Angiotensin Converting Enzyme (ACE) Inhibitors: Blood pressure medications that can cause chronic cough as a side effect. ACE inhibitors typically have generic names which end with the four letters "pril," for example: capto**pril**, mono**pril**, enalo**pril**.

Aspiration: The act of solid or liquid food going into the windpipe and lungs.

Barrett esophagus: A condition where stomach lining creeps up into its adjacent structure, the esophagus. Patients with Barrett have a 30–125 times greater chance of developing esophageal cancer than patients without Barrett.

Bronchoscopy: Examination of the lungs with a rigid or flexible camera.

Bronchoscope: An instrument that allows one to examine the windpipe (trachea) and lungs.

Carminatives: Substances that act to loosen the Lower Esophageal Sphincter (LES), the muscle that separates the stomach from the esophagus. Carminatives, such as onion and garlic, increase the chance of reflux of stomach acid into the esophagus and throat.

Conscious sedation: A type of "twilight" anesthesia which allows one to sedate patients without completely putting them to sleep, also known as intravenous sedation.

Diaphragm: The muscular structure that separates the stomach from the chest and lungs.

EsophagoGastroDuodenoscopy (EGD) (also known as **upper gastrointestinal (GI) endoscopy**): A method of examining the esophagus, stomach, and duodenum (upper portion of small intestine) almost always performed with the patient under conscious sedation.

Endoscope: A device that has a camera on one end that allows one to examine internal organs of the body. For example, a nasal endoscope allows a physician to examine the inside of the nose.

Endoscopy: A way of examining the inside of the body using a rigid or flexible instrument that has a camera either attached to it or embedded within the instrument.

Endosheath®: A single use, disposable sheath that completely covers the insertion tube of an endoscope. Think of it as a "condom" for an endoscope.

Esophageal adenocarcinoma: The type of esophageal cancer caused by acid reflux disease. The word "adeno" refers to "glands" as in mucus producing glands that line the esophagus.

Esophageal squamous cell carcinoma: The type of esophageal cancer typically caused by smoking cigarettes and drinking alcohol. The word "squamous" refers to the "skin," or lining of the esophagus.

Esophagitis: Inflammation of the esophagus.

Esophagram (also known as **Barium Swallow**): An X-ray test of the esophagus whereby a patient is given a sip of Barium while an X-ray is taken just as the patient is swallowing the barium.

Esophagus: A long, thin muscular tube that connects the throat to the stomach. It is where food travels from the throat to the stomach.

Fiberoptic Endoscopic Evaluation of Swallowing (FEES): A method of diagnosing swallowing problems by using a very thin flexible camera, placed via the nose, to observe the tongue, throat, vocal folds, windpipe and upper esophagus, while the patient is swallowing solid and liquid food.

Flexible Endoscopic Evaluation of Swallowing with Sensory Testing (FEESST): A method of diagnosing swallowing problems and assessing sensation in the throat by using a very thin flexible camera, placed via the nose, to observe the tongue, throat, vocal folds, windpipe and upper esophagus, while the patient is swallowing solid and liquid food.

Gastroenterologist (also known as a **Gastrointestinal (GI) doctor**): A doctor who specializes in treating diseases of the esophagus, stomach, intestines, and bowels.

Gastroenterology: The study of the science of digestion and the anatomy and physiology of the esophagus, stomach, intestines, and bowels.

Gastrointestinal (GI): Relating to the stomach and intestines (or bowel).

Gastro Esophageal Reflux Disease (GERD) (also known as **Heartburn Reflux**): A disease of the stomach and esophagus characterized by acid injury to these structures.

General anesthesia: Complete anesthesia where the patient is put to sleep for the duration of a surgical procedure. With general anesthesia the patient usually has a breathing tube inserted into their windpipe so their breathing is controlled by the person giving the anesthesia (anesthesiologist).

Granuloma: A benign growth that typically represents the body's response to chronic inflammation. For example, a vocal fold granuloma is the body's response to chronic acid reflux injury to the larynx or vocal folds.

Heartburn: The sensation of burning or irritation in the stomach and chest caused by stomach acid.

Hiatal hernia: An anatomic condition in which a portion of the stomach sits above the diaphragm (the muscular structure that separates the stomach from the chest and lungs).

Histamine-2 Receptor Antagonist (H2RA): A relatively short-acting antacid medication that prevents acid production in the stomach. Examples include famotidine (Pepcid), nizatidine (Axid), and ranitidine (Zantac).

Intravenous: Placing a substance in the vein, typically the primary method anesthesia is administered for upper and lower endoscopy.

Laryngologist: A doctor who specializes in treating both swallowing disorders as well as diseases of the vocal folds or larynx.

Laryngology: The study of voice and swallowing disorders, including diseases of the vocal folds, throat, and swallowing mechanisms.

Laryngopharyngeal: The vocal folds and throat.

LaryngoPharyngeal Reflux (LPR) (also known as **Silent Reflux** or **Throatburn Reflux**): Acid reflux disease affecting the voice, throat, vocal folds, and swallowing muscles.

Laryngoscope: A rigid or flexible camera that allows the examination of the larynx or vocal folds.

Laryngoscopy: Examination of the larynx with a rigid or flexible camera.

Larynx: The organ that contains the vocal folds.

Lower Esophageal Sphincter (LES): Anatomic muscular region of the lowest portion of the esophagus that separates the stomach from the esophagus. The structure that prevents stomach acid from flowing freely back up into the esophagus.

Macronutrients: Nutrients, such a proteins, fats, and carbohydrates that the body uses in relatively large amounts.

Micronutrients: Vitamins, minerals, and other trace elements which are vitally important, and are used by the body in relatively small amounts.

Modified Barium Swallow: An X-ray test of swallowing where the patient is given a cookie that is laced with Barium while an X-ray is taken just as the patient is swallowing the barium. This test looks at the entire mouth and throat swallowing mechanism including the lips, tongue, throat, larynx, windpipe, and top of the esophagus. It is the X-ray equivalent of a FEES or FEESST.

Otolaryngology: The study of anatomy, function, and diseases of the ear, nose, and throat.

Otolaryngologist (also known as an **Ear, Nose, and Throat doctor** or an **ENT doctor**): A doctor and surgeon who specializes in treating diseases of the ear, nose, and throat.

Paradoxical Vocal Fold Movement Disorder (PVFMD) (also known as **Vocal Cord Dysfunction (VCD)**): A disorder of unknown etiology (it is unknown what causes this disorder) where the vocal folds, instead of only slightly opening and closing during quiet breathing, stay completely closed or nearly closed.

Pepsin: An enzyme released by the stomach whose primary function is to break down protein. Pepsin is most active in an environment that has a pH level between 1-4 and becomes progressively less active at pH 5 or greater.

pH: Measurement of the acid or alkaline content of any substance. A neutral pH is 7.0, an acidic pH is less than 7 with the most acidic substance at a pH of 1. An alkaline pH is greater than 7 with the most alkaline substance at a pH of 14.

Proton Pump Inhibitor (PPI): A relatively long acting, potent antacid medication that prevents acid production in the stomach. Examples include dexlansoprazole (Dexilant), esomeprazole (Nexium), lansoprazole (Prevacid), omeprazole (Prilosec), omeprazole/sodium carbonate (Zegerid), pantoprazole (Protonix), rabeprazole (Aciphex).

Pulmonologist: A doctor who specializes in treating diseases of the lung.

Reflux: The backflow of any substance. Acid reflux refers to the back flow of, typically, stomach acid from its natural location in the stomach up to the esophagus or throat.

Regurgitation: The act of partially digested solid and/or liquid food from the stomach travelling up towards the chest and mouth.

Respiratory retraining: Increased resistance breathing exercises, generally administered by a speech language pathologist (speech therapist), used to treat patients with chronic cough due to Vocal Cord Dysfunction (VCD), or Paradoxical Vocal Fold Movement Disorder (PVFMD).

Sensory testing: A method of measuring sensation in the throat whereby pulses of air are delivered to the throat in order to elicit a vocal fold closing reflex.

Silent Reflux (also known as **Throatburn Reflux** or **LaryngoPharyngeal Reflux (LPR)**): Acid reflux without the patient complaining of heartburn and or regurgitation, but is complaining of a variety of throat symptoms.

Stroboscopy (also known as **Laryngeal Video Stroboscopy**): Examination of the larynx or vocal folds with a rigid or flexible camera that has a strobe light flashing light through it. The strobe light allows the rapidly vibrating vocal folds to dramatically slow down their vibrations so the examiner can see every detail of the vocal fold surface and how the vocal folds are vibrating.

Spirometer: A device that measures the amount, or volume, and speed of air that can be inhaled and exhaled during breathing.

Spirometry: A type of lung function test, or pulmonary function test, that measures the amount, or volume, and speed of air that can be inhaled and exhaled during breathing.

Throatburn Reflux (also known as **LPR** or **Silent Reflux**): Acid reflux with the patient complaining of throat symptoms such as cough, hoarseness, lump-like sensation in the throat, swallowing difficulty, and/or throat burning. The patient generally does not have heartburn or regurgitation.

TransNasal Esophagoscopy (TNE): A method of examining the esophagus by placing a thin, spaghetti-like camera through the nose then into the esophagus. It does not require sedation of any sort.

Transnasal Flexible Laryngoscopy (TFL): A method of examining the throat, larynx (or vocal folds), and base of the tongue with a thin, flexible camera that is placed via the nose.

Transnasal Flexible Laryngoscopy (TFL) and **Biopsy (TFL Biopsy):** A method of taking a sample of tissue from the throat, larynx (or vocal folds), and base of the tongue with an instrument that is passed through a thin, flexible camera that is placed via the nose.

Trachea: Windpipe.

Transnasal: Through the nose.

Transoral: Through the mouth.

Upper Esophageal Sphincter (UES): Anatomic muscular region of the highest portion of the esophagus that separates the throat from the esophagus. The structure that prevents back flow of material from the esophagus into the throat and lungs.

Vagus Nerve: One of the 12 cranial nerves (nerves originating in the brain) that control voice, vocal fold movement, and swallowing. Also known as the tenth cranial nerve.

Vocal cords: See **"Vocal folds"** below.

Vocal folds: Paired vibrating folds of tissue that produce sound when air passes between them; also known as **vocal cords.**

Vocal fold paralysis (also known as **vocal *cord* paralysis**): Completely impaired movement of the vocal folds. Since there are two vocal folds, right and left, vocal fold paralysis can involve one side or both sides of the vocal folds.

Vocal fold paresis (also known as **vocal *cord* paresis**): Partially, as opposed to completely, impaired movement of the vocal folds. Since there are two vocal folds, right and left, vocal fold paresis can involve one side or both sides of the vocal folds.

Z-line: Anatomic location that represents the transition between the bottom of the esophagus and the top of the stomach.

Zenker's diverticulum: A small pouch, or herniation (think of a kangaroo pouch), of the upper portion of the esophagus, where solid and liquid food can collect while eating and drinking. Since a Zenker's diverticulum is located so close to the larynx, when the pouch fills with solids or liquids, it can suddenly empty its contents right near the larynx, increasing chance of aspiration (solid or liquid material going into the windpipe).

SOURCES

*"The most remarkable thing about my mother is that
for thirty years she served the family nothing but leftovers.
The original meal has never been found."*

—CALVIN TRILLIN

CHAPTER ONE: ACID REFLUX DISEASE–THE MASTER OF DISGUISE

Bittman, M. (2009). Food Matters: A Guide to Conscious Eating. New York, NY: Simon & Schuster.

Cooper, A., Holmes, L.M. (2000). Bitter Harvest: A Chef's Perspective on the Hidden Dangers in the Foods We Eat and What You Can Do About It. New York, NY: Routledge.

Moss, M. (2013). Salt Sugar Fat: How the Food Giants Hooked Us. New York, NY: Random House.

Pohl, H., Welch, H.G. (2005). The role of over-diagnosis and reclassification in the marked increase of esophageal adenocarcinoma incidence. *Journal of the National Cancer Institute, 97(2):* 142–146.

Pollan, M. (2006). The Omnivore's Dilemma: A Natural History of Four Meals. New York, NY: The Penguin Press.

U.S. Food and Drug Administration. (2012). Draft Guidance for Industry: Acidified Foods. Food and Drug Administration. Retrieved from: http://www.fda.gov/Food/GuidanceComplianceRegulatoryInformation/GuidanceDocuments/AcidifiedandLow-AcidCannedFoods/ucm222618.htm

Langevin, S.M., Michaud, D.S., Marsit, C.J., Nelson, H.H., Birnbaum, A.E., Eliot, M., Christensen, B.C., McClean, M.D., Kelsey, K.T. (2013). Gastric reflux is an independent risk factor for laryngopharyngeal carcinoma. *Cancer Epidemiology, Biomarkers and Prevention, 22(6):* 1–8.

Thrift, A.P., Whiteman, D.C. (2012). The incidence of esophageal adenocarcinoma continues to rise: Analysis of period and birth cohort effects on recent trends. *Annals of Oncology, 23(12):* 3155-3162.

CHAPTER TWO: THE STOMACH IS CONNECTED TO THE THROAT

Aviv, J.E., Murry, T. (2005). FEESST (Flexible Endoscopic Evaluation of Swallowing with SensoryTesting). San Diego, CA: Plural Publishing Co.

Cook, I.J., Dodds, W.J., Dantas, R.O., Massey, B., Kern, M.K., Lang, M.M., Brasseur, J.G., Hogan, W.J. (1989). Opening mechanisms of the human upper esophageal sphincter. *American Journal of Physiology: Gastrointestinal and Liver Physiology, 257:* G748–G759.

Dent, J., Holloway, R.H., Toouli, J., Dodds, W.J.(1988). Mechanisms of lower oesophageal sphincter incompetence in patients with symptomatic gastrooesophageal reflux. *Gut, 29(8):* 1020–1028.

Edgren, G., Adami, H-O., Vaino, E.W., Nyren, O. (2013). A global assessment of the oesophageal adenocarcinoma epidemic. *Gut, 62:* 1406–1414.

Enzmann, D.R., Harell, G.S., Zboralske, F.F. (1977). Upper esophageal responses to intraluminal distention in man. *Gastroenterology, 72:* 1292–1298.

Holloway, R.H. (2000). Esophageal body motor response to reflux events: Secondary peristalsis. *American Journal of Medicine, 108:* S20–S26.

Kahrilas, P.J. (1997). Upper esophageal sphincter function during antegrade and retrograde transit. *American Journal of Medicine, 103:* 56S–60S.

Kern, M.K., Lang, M.M., Brasseur, J.G., Hogan, W.J. (1989). Opening mechanisms of the human upper esophageal sphincter. *American Journal of Physiology: Gastrointestinal and Liver Physiology, 257:* G748–G759.

Koufman, J.A., Aviv, J.E., Casiano, R.R., Shaw, G.Y. (2002). Laryngopharyngeal reflux: Position statement of the Committee on Speech, Voice, and Swallowing Disorders of the American Academy of Otolaryngology-Head and Neck Surgery. *Otolaryngology–Head and Neck Surgery, 127:* 32–35.

Lang, I.M., Medda, B.K., Shaker, R. (2001). Mechanisms of reflexes induced by esophageal distension. *American Journal of Physiology: Gastrointestinal and Liver Physiology, 281:* G1246–G1263.

Lohsiriwat, S., Puengna, N., Leelakusolvong, S. (2006). Effect of caffeine on lower esophageal sphincter pressure in Thai healthy volunteers. *Diseases of the Esophagus, 19(3):* 183-8.

Postma, G.N., Belafsky, P.C., Aviv, J.E. (2006). Atlas of Transnasal Esophagoscopy. Philadelphia, PA: Lippincott, Williams & Wilkins.

Schoeman, M.N., Holloway, R.H. (1994). Stimulation and characteristics of secondary esophageal peristalsis in normal subjects. *Gut, 35:* 152–158.

Shaker, R., Hogan, W.J. (2003). Normal physiology of aerodigestive tract and its effect on the upper gut. *American Journal of Medicine, 115:* 2S–9S.

Shaker, R., Ren, J., Xie, P., Lang, I.M., Bardan, E., Sui, Z. (1997). Characterization of the pharyngo-UES contractile reflex in humans. *American Journal of Physiology: Gastrointestinal and Liver Physiology, 273:* G854–G858.

Ulualp, S.O., Toohill, R.J., Kern, M., Shaker, R. (1988). Pharyngo-UES contractile reflex in patients with posterior laryngitis. *Laryngoscope, 108:* 1354–1357.

CHAPTER THREE: SILENT REFLUX: IT'S THROATBURN *NOT* HEARTBURN

Aviv, J.E. (1997). Sensory discrimination in the larynx and hypopharynx. *Otolaryngology-Head and Neck Surgery, 116:* 331-334.

Aviv, J.E., Mohr, J.P., Blitzer, A., Thomson, J., Close, L.G. (1997). Restoration of laryngopharyngeal sensation by neural anastomosis. *Archives of Otolaryngology-Head and Neck Surgery, 123:* 154-160.

Aviv, J.E., Kim, T., Thomson, J., Sunshine, S., Kaplan, S., Close, L.G. (1998). Fiberoptic endoscopic evaluation of swallowing with sensory testing (FEESST) in healthy controls, *Dysphagia, 13:* 87-92.

Aviv, J.E., Kim, T., Goodhart, K., Kaplan, S., Thomson, J., Diamond, B., Close, L.G. (1998). FEESST: A new bedside endoscopic test of the motor and sensory components of swallowing. *Annals of Otology, Rhinology, and Laryngology, 107:* 378-387.

Aviv, J.E. (1999). Endoscopic diagnosis of swallowing disturbance. *The Journal of Japan Society for Laser Surgery and Medicine, 20:* 169-188.

Aviv, J.E., Martin, J.H., Kim, T., Sacco, R.L., Thomson, J.E., Diamond, B., Close, L.G. (1999). Laryngopharyngeal sensory discrimination testing and the laryngeal adductor reflex. *Annals of Otology, Rhinology, and Laryngology, 108:* 725-730.

Aviv, J.E., Kim, T., Goodhart, K., Kaplan, S., Diamond, B., Close, L.G. (2000). The safety of flexible endoscopic evaluation of swallowing with sensory testing (FEESST): An analysis of 500 consecutive evaluations. *Dysphagia, 15:* 39-44.

Aviv, J.E. (2000). Clinical assessment of pharyngolaryngeal sensitivity. *American Journal of Medicine, 108(4A):* 68S-72S.

Aviv, J.E. (2000). Prospective, randomized outcome study of endoscopy versus modified barium swallow in patients with dysphagia. *Laryngoscope, 110:* 563-574.

Aviv, J.E., Liu, H., Parides, M., Kaplan, S.T., Close, L.G. (2000). Laryngopharyngeal sensory deficits in patients with laryngopharyngeal reflux and dysphagia. *Annals of Otology, Rhinology, and Laryngology, 109:* 1000-1006.

Aviv, J.E., Spitzer, J., Cohen, M., Ma, G., Belafsky, P.C., Close, L.G. (2002). Laryngeal adductor reflex and pharyngeal squeeze as predictors of laryngeal penetration and aspiration. *Laryngoscope, 112:* 338-341.

Aviv, J.E., Murry, T., Zschommler, A., Cohen, M., Gartner, C. (2005). Flexible Endoscopic Evaluation of Swallowing with Sensory Testing (FEESST): Patient characteristics and analysis of safety in 1340 consecutive examinations. *Annals of Otology, Rhinology, and Laryngology, 114:* 173-176.

Belafsky, P.C., Postma, G.N., Koufman, J.A. (2002). Validity and reliability of the reflux symptom index (RSI). *Journal of Voice, 16(2):* 274-277.

Koufman, J.A. (1991). The otolaryngologic manifestations of gastroesophageal reflux disease (GERD): A clinical investigation of 225 patients using ambulatory 24- hour pH monitoring and an experimental investigation of the role of acid and pepsin in the development of laryngeal injury. *Laryngoscope, 101(4 Pt 2 suppl 53):* 1-78.

Postma G.N., Belafsky P.C., Aviv J.E., Koufman J.A. (2002). Laryngopharyngeal reflux testing. *Ear Nose and Throat Journal, 81(suppl 2):* 14–18.

Sharma, P. (2009). Barrett's Esophagus. *New England Journal of Medicine, 361:* 2548–2556.

CHAPTER FOUR: COUGH IT UP! COUGH AND THROATBURN REFLUX

Altman, K., Irwin, R. (eds.). (2010). Cough: An Interdisciplinary Problem. *Otolaryngologic Clinics of North America, 43:* 1–220.

Endoh, K., Leung, F.W. (1994). Effects of smoking and nicotine on the gastric mucosa: A review of clinical and experimental evidence. *Gastroenterology, 107(3):* 864–78.

Ing, A.J., Ngu, M.C., Breslin, A.B. (1992). Chronic persistent cough and clearance of esophageal acid. *Chest, 102(6):* 1668–1671.

Irwin, R.S., Curley, F.J., French, C.L. (1990). Chronic cough. The spectrum and frequency of causes, key components of the diagnostic evaluation, and outcome of specific therapy. *American Review of Respiratory Disease, 141(3):* 640–647.

Kollarik, M., Brozmanova, M. (2009). Cough and gastroesophageal reflux: Insights from animal models. *Pulmonary Pharmacology and Therapeutics, 22(2):* 130–134.

Palombini, B.C., Villanova, C.A., Araújo, E., Gastal, O.L., Alt, D.C., Stolz, D.P., Palombini, C.O. (1999). A pathogenic triad in chronic cough: Asthma, postnasal drip syndrome, and gastroesophageal reflux disease. *Chest, 116(2):* 279–284.

Rattan, S., Goyal, R.K. (1975). Effect of nicotine on the lower esophageal sphincter. Studies on the mechanism of action. *Gastroenterology, 69(1):* 154–9.

Smith, J., Woodcock, A., Houghton, L. (2010). New developments in reflux-associated cough. *Lung, 188(suppl 1):* 81–86.

Sifrim, D., Dupont, L., Blondeau, K., Zhang, X., Tack, J., Janssens, J. (2005). Weakly acidic reflux in patients with chronic unexplained cough during 24 hour pressure, pH, and impedance monitoring. *Gut, 54(4):* 449–454.

CHAPTER FIVE: ESOPHAGEAL CANCER PREVENTION: TARGETING THE RIGHT SYMPTOMS

Aviv, J.E., Takoudes, T.G., Ma, G., Close, L.G. (2001). Office-based esophagoscopy: A preliminary report. *Otolaryngology–Head and Neck Surgery, 125:* 170–5.

Aviv, J.E. (2006). Transnasal esophagoscopy: State of the art. *Otolaryngology–Head and Neck Surgery, 135:* 616–619.

Amin, M.R., Postma, G.N., Setzen, M., Koufman, J.A. (2008). Transnasal esophagoscopy: A position statement from the American Bronchoesophagological Association (ABEA). *Otolaryngology–Head and Neck Surgery, 138(4):* 411–4.

Bailey, P.L., Zuccaro, G. (2006). Sedation for endoscopic procedures: Not as simple as it seems. *American Journal of Gastroenterology, 101:* 2008–2010.

Belafsky, P.C., Postma, G.N., Daniel, E., Koufman, J.A. (2001). Transnasal esophagoscopy. *Otolaryngology-Head and Neck Surgery, 125(6):* 588–9.

Blondheim, D.S., Levi, D., Marmor, A.T. (2004). Mild sedation before transesophageal echo induces significant hemodynamic and respiratory depression. *Echocardiography, 21(3):* 241–245.

Carter, K.C., Carter, B.R. (1994). Childbed Fever: A Scientific Biography of Ignaz Semmelweis. Westport, CT: Greenwood Publishing Group.

Catanzaro, A., Faulx, A., Isenberg, G.A., Wong, R.K.C., Cooper, G., Sivak, M.V., Chak, A. (2003). Prospective evaluation of 4 mm diameter endoscopes for esophagoscopy in sedated and unsedated patients. *Gastrointestinal Endoscopy, 57:* 300–4.

Center for Disease Control and Prevention. Handwashing: Clean hands save lives. Retrieved from www.cdc.gov/handwashing/

Center for Disease Control and Prevention. (2002, October). Guideline for hand hygiene in health-care settings: Recommendations of the Healthcare Infection Control Practices Advisory Committee and the HICPAC/SHEA/APIC/IDSA Hand Hygiene Task Force. *Morbidity and Mortality Weekly Report, 51:* 1–45.

Chamberlain, G. (2006). British maternal mortality in the 19th and early 20th centuries. *Journal of Royal Society of Medicine, 99(11):* 559–563.

Cohen, L.B., DeLegge, M.H., Aisenberg, J., Brill, J.V., Inadomi, J.M., Kochman, M.L., Piorkowski, J.D. (2007). AGA Institute review of endoscopic sedation. *Gastroenterology, 133:* 675–701.

Eloubeidi, M.A., Provenzale, D. (2001). Clinical and demographic predictors of Barrett's esophagus among patients with gastroesophageal reflux disease: A multivariable analysis in veterans. *Journal of Clinical Gastroenterology, 33(4):* 306–309.

Falcone, M.T., Garrett, C.G., Slaughter, J.C., Vaezi, M. (2009). Transnasal esophagoscopy findings: Interspecialty comparison. *Otolaryngology-Head and Neck Surgery, 140(6):* 812–815.

Faulx, A.L., Catanzaro, A., Zyzanski, S., Cooper, G.S., Pfau, P.R., Isenberg, G., Wong, R.C.K., Sivak, M.V., Chak, A. (2002). Patient tolerance and acceptance of unsedated ultrathin endoscopy. *Gastrointestinal Endoscopy, 55:* 620–623.

Gerstenberger, P.D., Plumeri, P.A. (1993). Malpractice claims in gastrointestinal endoscopy: Analysis of an insurance industry data base. *Gastrointestinal Endoscopy, 39:* 132–8.

Hallett, C. (2005). The attempt to understand puerperal fever in the eighteenth and early nineteenth centuries: The influence of inflammation theory. *Medical History, 49:* 1–28.

Jackson, C. (1938). The Life of Chevalier Jackson: An Autobiography. New York, NY: Macmillan.

Jobe, B.A., Hunter, J.G., Chang, E.Y., Kim, C.Y., Eisen, G.M., Robinson, J.D., Diggs, B.S., O'Rourke, R.W., Rader, A.E., Schipper, P., Sauer, D.A., Peters, J.H., Lieberman, D.A., Morris, C.D. (2006). Office-based unsedated small-caliber endoscopy is equivalent to conventional sedated endoscopy in screening and surveillance for Barrett's esophagus: A randomized and blinded comparison. *American Journal of Gastroenterology, 101*: 2693–703.

Locke, G.R., Zinsmeister, A.R., Talley, N.J. (2003). Can symptoms predict endoscopic findings in GERD? *Gastrointestinal Endoscopy, 58(5):* 661–670.

McQuaid, K.R., Laine, L. (2008). A systematic review and meta-analysis of randomized, controlled trials of moderate sedation for routine endoscopic procedures. *Gastrointestinal Endoscopy, 67(6):* 910–923.

Mokhashi, M.S., Wildi, S.M., Glenn, T.F., Wallace, M.B., Jost, C., Gumustop, B., Kim, C.Y., Cotton, P.B., Hawes, R.H. (2003). A prospective, blinded study of diagnostic esophagoscopy with a superthin, stand-alone, battery-powered esophagoscope. *American Journal of Gastroenterology, 98:* 2383–2389.

Nason, K.S, Wichienkuer, P.P., Awais, O., Schuchert, M.J., Luketich, J.D., O'Rourke, R.W., Hunter, J.G., Morris, C.D., Jobe, B.A. (2011). Gastroesophageal reflux disease symptom severity, proton pump inhibitor use, and esophageal carcinogenesis. *Archives of Surgery, 146(7):* 851–8.

Niemantsverdriet, E., Timmer, R., Breumelhof, R., Smout, A.J.P.M. (1997). The roles of excessive gastro-oesophageal reflux, disordered oesophageal motility and decreased mucosal sensitivity in the pathogenesis of Barrett's oesophagus. *European Journal of Gastroenterology and Hepatology, 9(5):* 515–519.

Prescott, C.A. (1993). Outpatient pediatric oesophagoscopy using a flexible fibreoptic bronchoscope. Design of an insufflation-aspiration adaptor. *International Journal of Pediatric Otorhinolaryngology, 27(2):* 113–118.

Petrini, J., Egan, J.V. (2004). Risk management regarding sedation/analgesia. *Gastrointestinal Endoscopic Clinicians of North America, 14:* 401–414.

Postma, G., Cohen, J., Belafsky, P., Halum, S., Gupta, S., Bach, K., Koufman, J. (2005). Transnasal esophagoscopy: Revisited (over 700 consecutive cases). *Laryngoscope, 115:* 321–323.

Reavis, K.M., Morris, C.D., Gopal, D.V., Hunter, J.G., Jobe, B.A. (2004). Laryngopharyngeal reflux symptoms better predict the presence of esophageal adenocarcinoma than typical gastroesophageal reflux symptoms. *Annals of Surgery, 239:* 849–858.

Shaker, R. (1994). Unsedated trans-nasal pharyngoesophagogastroduodenoscopy (T-EGD): Technique. *Gastrointestinal Endoscopy, 40(3):* 346–348.

Saeian, K., Staff, D., Vasilopoulos, S., Townsend, W. F., Almagro, U.A., Komorowski, R. A., Choi, H., Shaker, R. (2002). Unsedated transnasal endoscopy accurately detects Barrett's metaplasia and dysplasia. *Gastrointestinal Endoscopy, 56:* 472–478.

Thota, P.N., Zuccaro, G., Vargo, J.J., Conwell, D.L., Dumot, J.A., Xu, M. (2005). A randomized prospective trial comparing unsedated esophagoscopy via transnasal and transoral routes using a 4-mm video endoscope with conventional endoscopy with sedation. *Endoscopy, 37:* 559-565.

Zaman, A., Hahn, M., Hapke, R., Knigge, K., Fennerty, M.B., Katon, R.M. (1999). A randomized trial of peroral versus transnasal endoscopy using ultrathin video endoscope. *Gastrointestinal Endoscopy, 49:* 279-84.

CHAPTER SIX: THE BUILDING BLOCKS OF THE ACID WATCHER® DIET: HOW CARBOHYDRATES, PROTEINS, AND FATS AFFECT OUR BODIES

Basson, M. (2002). Gut mucosal healing: Is the science relevant? *Americal Journal of Pathology, 161(4):* 1101-1105.

Berry, W., Pollan, M. (2009). Bringing It To The Table: On Farming and Food. Berkeley, CA: Counterpoint Press.

Donaghue, K.C., Pena, M.M., Chan, A.K.F., Blades, B.L., King, J., Storlien, L.H., Silink, M. (2000). Beneficial effects of increasing monounsaturated fat intake in adolescents with type 1 diabetes. *Diabetes Research and Clinical Practice, 48:* 193-199.

Dukan, P. (2011). The Dukan Diet: 2 Steps to Lose the Weight, 2 Steps to Keep It Off Forever. New York, NY: Crown Publishing Group.

El-Serag, H.B., Satia, J.A., Rabeneck, L. (2005). Dietary intake and the risk of gastro- esophageal reflux disease: A cross sectional study in volunteers. *Gut, 54(1):* 11-17.

Esselstyn, C. (2007). Prevent and Reverse Heart Disease: The Revolutionary, Scientifically Proven, Nutrition-Based Cure. New York, NY: The Penguin Group.

Gates, D., Schrecengost, L. (2011). The Baby Boomer Diet: Body Ecology's Guide to Growing Younger. New York, NY: Hay House Publishing.

Panel on Macronutrients, Panel on the Definition of Dietary Fiber, Subcommittee on Upper Reference Levels of Nutrients, Subcommittee on Interpretation and Uses of Dietary Reference Intakes, and the Standing Committee on the Scientific Evaluation of Dietary Reference Intakes, Food and Nutrition Board, Institute of Medicine of the National Academies. *Dietary reference intakes for energy, carbohydrate, fiber, fat, fatty acids, cholesterol, protein, and amino acids.* The National Academies Press. Washington, DC. 2005.

Rybicki, S. The Importance of HUFAs in Fish Food, Retrieved from: http://www.angelsplus.com/ArticleHufa.htm

Savarino, E., de Bortoli, N., Zentilin, P., Martinucci, I., Bruzzone, L., Furnari, M., Marchi, S., Savarino, V. (2012). Alginate controls heartburn in patients with erosive and nonerosive reflux disease. *World Journal of Gastroenterology, 18(32):* 4371-4378.

Simopoulos, A.P. (2008). The importance of the omega-6/omega-3 fatty acid ratio in cardiovascular disease and other chronic diseases. *Experimental Biology and Medicine, 233(6):* 674-88.

Taubes, G. (2007, July 7). What if it's all been a big fat lie? *The New York Times*. Retrieved from: http://www.nytimes.com/2002/07/07/magazine/what-if-it-is-all-been-a-big-fat-lie.html?pagewanted=all&src=pm

CHAPTER SEVEN: pH BASICS AND THE pH OF COMMONLY CONSUMED FOODS

Dwyer, J., Foulkes, E., Evans, M., Ausman, L. (1985). Acid/alkaline ash diets: Time for assessment and change. *Journal of American Dietetic Association, 85:* 841–845.

Frassetto, L., Morris, R.C., Sellmeyer, D.E., Todd, K., Sebastian, A. (2001). Diet, evolution and aging: The pathophysiologic effects of the post-agricultural inversion of the potassium-to-sodium and base-to-chloride ratios in the human diet. *European Journal of Nutrition, 40(5):* 200–13.

Johnston, N., Knight, J., Dettmar, P.W., Lively, M.O., Koufman, J. (2004). Pepsin and carbonic anhydrase isoenzyme III as diagnostic markers for laryngopharyngeal reflux disease. *Laryngoscope, 114:* 2129–34.

Johnston, N., Dettmar, P.W., Bishwokarma, B., Lively, M.O., Koufman, J.A. (2007). Activity/stability of human pepsin: implications for reflux attributed laryngeal disease. *Laryngoscope, 117:* 1036–9.

Myers, R.J. (2010). One hundred years of pH. *Journal of Chemical Education, 87:* 30–32.

Remer, T. (2000). Influence of diet on acid-base balance. *Seminars in Dialysis, 13(4):* 221–226.

Schwalfenberg, G. (2012). The alkaline diet: Is there evidence that an alkaline pH diet benefits health? *Journal of Environmental and Public Health,* Article ID 727630. doi:10.1155/2012/727630

U.S. Food and Drug Administration. (2007). Approximate pH of Foods and Food Products. Retrieved from: http://www.foodscience.caes.uga.edu/extension/documents/fdaapproximatephoffoodslacf-phs.pdf

Vyas, B., Le Quesne, S. (2007). The pH Balance Diet: Restore Your Acid-Alkaline Levels to Eliminate Toxins and Lose Weight. Berkeley, CA: Ulysses Press.

Young, R., Young, S. (2010). The pH Miracle for Weight Loss: Balance Your Body Chemistry, Achieve Your Ideal Weight. New York, NY: Grand Central Publishing, Hachette Publishing Group.

CHAPTER EIGHT: DR. AVIV'S ACID WATCHER® DIET: A DIET YOU CAN LIVE BY

Aviv, J.E., Liu, H., Parides, M., Kaplan, S.T., Close, L.G. (2000). Laryngopharyngeal sensory deficits in patients with laryngopharyngeal reflux and dysphagia. *Annals of Otology, Rhinology, and Laryngology, 109:* 1000–1006.

Aggarwal, B.B., Prasad, S., Reuter, S., Kannappan, R., Yadev, V.R., Park, B., Kim, J.H., Gupta, S.C., Phromnoi, K., Sundaram, C., Prasad, S., Chaturvedi, M.M., Sung, B. (2011). Identification of novel anti-inflammatory agents from Ayurvedic medicine for prevention of chronic diseases "Reverse Pharmacology" and "Bedside to Bench" approach. *Current Drug Targets, 12(11):* 1595-1653.

Campbell, T.M., Campbell, T.C. (2004). The China Study: The Most Comprehensive Study of Nutrition Ever Conducted and the Startling Implications for Diet, Weight Loss and Long-Term Health. Dallas, TX: BenBella Books.

Chung, M.Y., Lim, T.G., Lee, K.W. (2013). Molecular mechanisms of chemopreventive phytochemicals against gastroenterological cancer development. *World Journal of Gastroenterology, 19(7):* 984-93.

Coleman, H.G., Murray, L.J., Hicks, B., Bhat, S.K., Kubo, A., Corley, D.A., Cardwell, C.R., Cantwell, M.M. (2013). Dietary fiber and the risk of precancerous lesions and cancer of the esophagus: A systematic review and meta-analysis. *Nutrition Reviews, 71(7):* 474-82.

Kubo, A., Levin, T.R., Block, G., Rumore, G.J., Quesenberry, C.P., Buffler, P., Corley, D.A. (2008). Dietary antioxidants, fruits, and vegetables and the risk of Barrett's esophagus. *American Journal of Gastroenterology, 103(7):* 1614-23.

Lustig, R. H. (2013) Fat Chance: Beating the Odds Against Sugar, Processed Food, Obesity, and Disease. New York, NY: Hudson Street Press.

Massey, B.T. (2001). Diffuse esophageal spasm: A case for carminatives? *Journal of Clinical Gastroenterology, 33(1):* 8-10.

Pollan, M. (2008). In Defense of Food: An Eater's Manifesto. New York, NY: The Penguin Press.

Watson, B., Smith, L. (2007). The Fiber35 Diet: Nature's Weight Loss Secret. New York, NY: Simon & Schuster.

APPENDIX A

Aviv, J.E., Johnson, L.F. (2000). Flexible endoscopic evaluation of swallowing with sensory testing (FEESST) to diagnose and manage patients with pharyngeal dysphagia. *Practical Gastroenterology, 24:* 52-59.

Aviv, J.E., Parides, M., Fellowes, J., Close, L.G. (2000). Endoscopic evaluation of swallowing as an alternative to 24-hour pH monitoring to diagnose extra-esophageal reflux. *Annals of Otology, Rhinology, and Laryngology, 109(suppl.184):* 25-27.

Harding, S.M., Richter, J.E. (1997). The role of gastroesophageal reflux in chronic cough and asthma. *Chest, 111:* 1389-1402.

Lee, B., Woo, P. (2005). Chronic cough as a sign of laryngeal sensory neuropathy: Diagnosis and treatment. *Annals of Otology, Rhinology, and Laryngology, 114:* 253-257.

Mishriki, Y.Y. (2007). Laryngeal neuropathy as a cause of chronic intractable cough. *American Journal of Medicine, 120:* 5-7.

Phua, S.Y., McGarvey, L.P.A., Ngu, M.C., Ing, AJ. (2005). Patients with gastro-oesophageal reflux disease and cough have impaired laryngopharyngeal mechanosensitivity. *Thorax, 60:* 488–491.

APPENDIX B

Altman, K.W., Simpson, C.B., Amin, M.R., Abaza, M., Balkissoon, R., Casiano, R.R. (2002). Cough and paradoxical vocal fold motion. *Otolaryngology–Head and Neck Surgery, 127:* 501–511.

Christopher, K.L., Wood, R.P., Eckert, R.C., Blager, F.B., Raney, R.A., Souhrada, J.F. (1983). Vocal-cord dysfunction presenting as asthma. *New England Journal of Medicine, 308:* 1566–1570.

Morrison, M., Rammage, L., Emami, A.J. (1999). The irritable larynx syndrome. *Journal of Voice, 13:* 447–455.

Mintz S, Lee, J.K. (2006). Gabapentin in the treatment of intractable chronic cough: Case reports. *American Journal of Medicine, 119:* 13–15.

Murry, T., Tabaee, A., Aviv, J.E. (2004). Respiratory retraining of refractory cough and laryngopharyngeal reflux in patients with paradoxical vocal fold movement disorder. *Laryngoscope, 114:* 1341–1345

Murry, T., Tabaee, A., Owczarzak, V., Aviv, J.E. (2006). Respiratory retraining therapy and management of laryngopharyngeal reflux in the treatment of patients with cough and paradoxical vocal fold movement disorder. *Annals of Otology, Rhinology, and Laryngology, 115:* 754–758.

Murry, T., Sapienza, C. (2010). The role of voice therapy in the management of paradoxical vocal fold motion, chronic cough, and laryngospasm. *Otolaryngology Clinics of North America, 43:* 73–83.

Murry, T., Branski, R., Yu, K., Cukier-Blaj, S., Duflo, S., Aviv, J.E. (2010). Laryngeal sensory deficits in patients with chronic cough and paradoxical vocal fold movement disorder. *Laryngoscope, 120(8):* 1576–1581.

Newman, K.B., Mason, U.G., Schmaling, K.B. (1995). Clinical features of vocal cord dysfunction. *American Journal of Respiratory and Critical Care Medicine, 152:* 1382–1386.

Rogers, J.H, Stell, P.M. (1978). Paradoxical movement of the vocal cords as a cause of stridor. *Journal of Laryngology and Otology, 92:* 157–158.

Vertigan, A.E., Theodoros, D.G., Gibson, P.G., Winkworth, A.L. (2006). The relationship between chronic cough and paradoxical vocal fold movement: A review of the literature. *Journal of Voice, 20:* 466–480.

Wani, M.K., Woodson, G.E. (1999). Paroxysmal laryngospasm after laryngeal nerve injury. *Laryngoscope, 109:* 694–697.

ABOUT THE AUTHOR

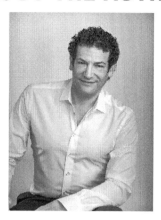

Dr. Jonathan E. Aviv, MD, FACS is the Clinical Director and founder of the Voice and Swallowing Center at ENT and Allergy Associates, LLP in New York City. He is also Clinical Professor of Otolaryngology, Icahn School of Medicine at Mount Sinai and an Attending Physician in The Mount Sinai Hospital in New York. Dr. Aviv is the former Director, Division of Head and Neck Surgery, Department of Otolaryngology-Head and Neck Surgery, College of Physicians and Surgeons, Columbia University.

He is the inventor and developer of the endoscopic air-pulse laryngeal sensory testing technology, known as FEESST. Dr. Aviv has authored over 60 scientific papers in peer-reviewed journals and has written two medical text books entitled *Flexible Endoscopic Evaluation of Swallowing with Sensory Testing (FEESST)* and *Atlas of Transnasal Esophagoscopy.*

Dr. Aviv is Past President of the American Broncho-Esophagological Association and the New York Laryngological Society, and former Chairman of the Speech, Voice and Swallowing Disorders Committee, American Academy of Otolaryngology-Head and Neck Surgery.

Dr. Aviv has been in *New York Magazine's* "Best Doctors" 1998–2013, *Best Doctors in America* 2004–2013, *Who's Who in America, Who's Who in Medicine and Healthcare* and *Who's Who in Science and Engineering.*

Dr. Aviv has written a blog for *The Dr. Oz Show* website and has been featured in press articles in the *New York Times* and the *Wall Street Journal.* He has also appeared on *Good Morning America, The Dr. Oz Show, Bloomberg Television,* and the *Discovery Channel.*

ACKNOWLEDGEMENTS

"Quality is not an act, it is a habit."
—ARISTOTLE

Just like no surgeon can perform an operation alone, no book is ever completed by a single individual.

A special thank you to my brother, Bobby Elijah Aviv, and sister-in-law, Giordona Aviv, without whom this book could never have been completed. They followed me through the process every step of the way. Their encouragement as well as contributions extend from the cover design to countless hours of editing. I owe particular gratitude to Giordona, who is a health and wellness expert, for her vital assistance in the realization of the Acid Watcher® Diet.

Many thanks go to my professional colleagues from my years at Columbia University, Drs. Andrew Blitzer, James Dillard, J.P. Mohr, Byron Thomashow, Lanny Close, Hector Rodriguez, Ian Storper, Herbert Pardes, and Steven Corwin. I am grateful to Florence and Herbert Irving for their largess and vision which enabled some of my original clinical research to be funded and carried out.

Much appreciation goes to Thomas Murry, SLP, PhD, the renowned speech language pathologist who worked side by side with me for 10 years at the Voice and Swallowing Center at Columbia. In addition, speech language pathologists Manderly Cohen, Carolyn Gartner, Winston Cheng, and Gaetano Fava were also extremely helpful from the outset of the FEESST training program at Columbia. A special thanks to Drs. Robert Ossoff, Stanley Shapshay, Charles Ford, and Steven Zeitels, who were extraordinarily supportive of TNE from its infancy and ran enough interference to allow ideas off the beaten path to nurture and eventually flourish.

I would like to thank all my colleagues, staff, and administration at ENT and Allergy Associates, LLP. In particular, my fellow laryngologists at the Voice and Swallowing Center, Drs. David Godin, Jared Wasserman, Farhad Chowdhury, Joel Portnoy, and Ajay Chitkara, have been instrumental in helping to broaden the breadth and depth of our Voice and Swallowing Center. I would also like to thank my partners in my clinical offices, Drs. Robert Green, Steven Sacks, Scott Markowitz, Guy Lin, Won Choe, Michael Bergstein, Jill Zeitlin, John County, and Lynelle Granady. Also, special thanks to Drs. Marc Levine and Moshe Ephrat. Further thanks to the Speech Language Pathologists at ENT and Allergy Associates, Christie Block, Amanda Hembree, Danielle Falciglia, and Heather Jones as well as my medical assistants Cosette Osmani and Charleen Male. The administrative team at ENT and Allergy Associates, in particular, Robert Glazer, Richard Effman, and Dr. Wayne Eisman, were very helpful and encouraging.

Much gratitude to my medical colleagues around the country for their support—Drs. Robert Sataloff, Dana Thompson, Marshall Strome, Michael Beninger, David Posner, Ken Altman, Eric Genden, Peak Woo, Peter Belafsky, Greg Postma, and Jamie Koufman.

The awareness of TNE overseas was greatly enhanced by Drs. Jean Abitbol, Gabriel Jaume, Manolo Tomas, and Peter Friedland.

I would like to thank the following gastroenterologists for their support and guidance—Drs. David Markowitz, Charles Lightdale, Jonathan LaPook, Stanley Benjamin, Phil Katz, Joel Richter, Reza Shaker, Alin Botoman, Michael Vaezi, Greg Haber, Robert Fath, and Sharmila Anandasabapathy.

Industry was critical in the transformation of ideas into reality, notably Lewis Pell, Katsumi Oneda, Nicholas Tsaclas, Ron Hadani, Mark Fletcher, Janis Saunier, David Damm, Ted Phelan, Alex Gorsky, Dr. Harlan Weisman, Bo Reilly, and Damion Michaels.

I am grateful to my friends and colleagues in the media and entertainment world who have brought attention to the dangers of untreated acid reflux, including Diane Sawyer, Dr. Mehmet Oz, Dr. Jay Adlersberg, Pimm Fox, Jane Brody, Carol Brodie, Ian Axel, Chris Barron, John Turturro, and Jack Rosenthal.

Thank you to my close friends Jonathan Rapillo, Cherish Gallant, Robert Berman, Jonathan Lowenberg, Marc Mazur, Jonathan Halpern, Eugene Carozza, Ira Kaufman, Herb Subin, and Paul Michael Weiner, for their encouragement and support as this project developed and unfolded.

My appreciation and gratitude to Harvey Shapiro for his excellent legal advice as well as his continued friendship over the years.

I would like to thank my editor, Kevin Anderson, who along with Bobby and Giordona Aviv, was instrumental in editing the book. My book designer, Tara Long, was an extraordinary help and talent as well. In addition to Giordona Aviv's work on the recipes, I would like to thank chefs Emiko Shimojo and Maureen Schreyer for contributing some of the recipes as well. I am also grateful to dieticians Diane Insolia, Melissa Kessler, and Anita Mirchandani.

A special thanks to my brother, Oren Aviv, for his support and encouragement and my parents, Rena and David Aviv, for their everlasting love and faith in all of my medical endeavors since the beginning of my career, when I first put a band-aid on my mother's elbow when I was six.

Finally, I would like to thank my patients. I hope that by the writing of this book, I will continue to reach out to those in need, through the expression of the ideas set forth in this book.

INDEX

Coffee, 5, 6, 15, 81, 135, 138, 140, 142-143, 145-147, 150, 157, 161, 164, 167-168, 175, 177, 180
Columbia University, 46, 173, 201
Columbia Presbyterian Medical Center, 2, 14, 17
Conscious Sedation, 39, 40, 42, 49
Cooper, Ann, 6
Cough, 3-4, 11, 16, 18-19, 21-25, 27-30, 33, 35, 38-39, 47, 49, 81, 133, 150-156, 169-178

Dr. Aviv Cough Algorithm, The, 26-28
Dr. Aviv Diet®, iv, 79, 183
Dr. Aviv Smoothie, 78, 82, 86, 90, 99
Dr. Oz Show, The, 30, 47, 201

Endoscopy, ix, 25, 39, 48-49, 133, 136, 150, 155-156, 161, 184, 185
ENT and Allergy Associates, 201
Esophageal Cancer, vi, xi,4, 5, 7-8, 17, 18, 20, 33-40, 46, 49, 54, 133-134, 183, 184
EsophagoGastroDuodenoscopy (EGD), 39, 40-42, 48-50, 156, 184
Evamor Water, 76

Fats, vii, 54, 63, 69, 186
    Monounsaturated, 64-65
    Omega-3, 65-67
    Omega-6, 65-67
    Polyunsaturated, 65-66
    Saturated, 62, 67-68
    Trans, 63-64
Fiberoptic Endoscopic Evaluation of Swallowing (FEES), 184, 186
Flexible Endoscopic Evaluation of Swallowing with Sensory Testing (FEESST), ix, 17-18, 40, 41,132-133, 157, 158, 161, 163, 165, 166,180,185, 186

Garrett, Gaelyn, 46
Gastro Esophageal Reflux Disease (GERD), 11, 16-17, 19, 20, 170, 172, 185
Good Morning America, 42, 47, 201
Granuloma, 146-150, 185

Handwashing, 35-37
Heartburn, vi, xi, 3-4, 11, 15, 16-21, 24, 29, 34-36, 38-39, 46-47, 71, 81, 133, 135, 138-139, 142, 145, 154-156, 159, 161, 163, 167, 185
Heartburn Reflux, 16-19, 20, 81, 144, 159, 170, 172, 185
Hiatal Hernia, 137, 152, 157, 167, 176, 181, 185

Pentax, 41-42

Pepsin, 72-73, 138, 141, 145, 187

Phytochemicals, 56

Pollan, Michael, 5, 183

Postma, Greg, 19, 46

Prescott, C.A., 41

Protein, 55, 61-62, 69, 72, 79, 85, 87, 111

Proton-Pump Inhibitors (PPI), 30-32, 136, 140, 143-144, 147-149, 151, 152, 164, 166, 168, 175-176, 178, 181-182, 187

Recipes, 90-121, 126-130

Regurgitation, 3-4, 19, 81, 133, 145, 154, 167-168

Rigid Esophagoscopy, 39

Semmelweis, Ignaz, 35-37

Setzen, Michael, 46

Shaker, Reza, 41

    Shaker exercises, 159-160

Silent Reflux, xi, 16-17, 188

Throatburn Reflux, vii, x, xi, 16-19, 21-22, 23-24, 27, 31-32, 37, 46-48, 81, 133, 135-136, 144, 153-154, 159, 164, 166, 168, 170, 172, 175-176, 180, 188

Thompson, Dana, 13-14

TIDE (Targeted Individual Diagnostic Effort), 37-38, 49, 134, 156

Title 21, 7-8

Trigger Foods, 81

TransNasal Esophagoscopy (TNE), 27, 38, 40-41, 133, 137, 140-141, 143, 147, 151-152, 167-168, 176, 181, 188

Tsaclas, Nicholas, 41-42

Upper Esophageal Sphincter (UES), 9, 11, 158-159, 189

Vision Sciences, 42

Vocal Folds, 12, 15, 21, 29-30, 72, 136-139, 142-144, 149, 151-152, 154, 158-159, 161, 169, 171-173, 175-176, 178, 180

Vocal Fold Paralysis, 27, 30

Vocal Cord Dysfunction (VCD), 27, 169-176, 178, 180, 181, 187

Z-line, 144, 147, 176, 181, 189

Zeitels, Steven, x